Public Health
in
America

This is a volume in the Arno Press series

PUBLIC HEALTH
IN
AMERICA

Advisory Editor

Barbara Gutmann Rosenkrantz

Editorial Board
**Leona Baumgartner
James H. Cassedy
Arthur Jack Viseltear**

See last pages of this volume
for a complete list of titles.

THE CARRIER STATE

ARNO PRESS

A New York Times Company

New York / 1977

Editorial Supervision: JOSEPH CELLINI

———◦◦◦———

The Work of a Chronic Typhoid Germ
    Distributor (Vol.48, No.24, June 15,1907,
    pp.2019-2022) and Typhoid Bacilli Carriers
    (Vol.51, No.12, September 19, 1908, pp.981-
    982), Copyright 1907-08, American Medical
    Association, were reprinted by permission
    of the American Medical Association.

PUBLIC HEALTH IN AMERICA
ISBN for complete set: 0-405-09804-9
See last pages of this volume for titles.

Manufactured in the United States of America

———◦◦◦———

Library of Congress Cataloging in Publication Data
Main entry under title:

The Carrier state.

    (Public health in America)
    Reprint of articles published 1895-1919.
    CONTENTS: Park, W. H. Report on bacteriological
investigations and diagnosis of diphtheria from May 4,
1893 to May 4, 1894.--Soper, G. The work of a chronic
typhoid germ distributor.--Park, W. H. Typhoid bacilli
carriers.--Soper, G. Typhoid Mary.
    1. Carrier state (Communicable diseases)--Addresses,
essays, lectures. 2. Typhoid fever--Transmission--
Addresses, essays, lectures. 3. Diphtheria--Transmission
--Addresses, essays, lectures. I. Park, William
Hallock, 1863-1939. II. Soper, George Albert, 1870-
1948. III. Series.
RA641.5.C37   614.5'112   76-40660
ISBN 0-405-09870-7

CONTENTS

SCIENTIFIC BULLETIN No. 1.

HEALTH DEPARTMENT, CITY OF NEW YORK,

From the Bacteriological Laboratory.

- - - - - - - -

REPORT

ON

BACTERIOLOGICAL INVESTIGATIONS

AND

DIAGNOSIS OF DIPHTHERIA.

From May 4, 1893, to May 4, 1894.

- - - - - - - -

HERMANN M. BIGGS, M. D.,

Pathologist and Director of the Bacteriological Laboratory.

WM. H. PARK, M. D.,

Bacteriological Diagnostician and Inspector of Diphtheria.

ALFRED L. BEEBE, PH. B.,

Inspector of Bacteriology

NEW YORK:

MARTIN B. BROWN, PRINTER AND STATIONER,

Nos. 49 TO 57 PARK PLACE.

———

1895.

November 9, 1953

To Members of the American Public Health Association
and their Guests:

In 1892, as the result of the cholera epidemic in Hamburg,
the City of New York established a bacteriological laboratory in
the Department of Health -- the first municipally operated public
health laboratory in the United States. After the cholera scare was
over, the laboratory, instead of being discontinued, began work on
the bacteriological examination of cultures for diphtheria.
William Hallock Park, M.D., was placed in charge of this work as
"Bacteriological Diagnostician and Inspector of Diphtheria."

The first scientific bulletin issued by the New York
City Department of Health, "A Report on Bacteriological
Investigations and Diagnosis of Diphtheria," by Doctor Park, has
been reproduced by the photo-offset process. It is being offered at
this 81st Annual Meeting of the American Public Health Association
in New York City in November, 1953, as a souvenir commemorating an
important date in public health.

It is fitting that Doctor Park's report on his original
investigations in the bacteriology of diphtheria be reissued by the
department in which he did his most outstanding work. It is equally
appropriate that we today make note of its publication, for it marks
the entrance of the Department of Health of the City of New York into
the field of scientific preventive medicine.

John F. Mahoney, M.D.
Commissioner

BACTERIOLOGICAL LABORATORY.

REPORT ON BACTERIOLOGICAL INVESTIGATIONS AND DIAGNOSIS OF DIPHTHERIA.

CHARLES F. ROBERTS, M. D., *Sanitary Superintendent :*

SIR—I have the honor to submit the following history and report of the bacteriological and experimental work on diphtheria performed in the Bacteriological Laboratory of the Health Department during the past year.

Early in January, 1893, a communication was addressed to the Board of Health of New York City, recommending the systematic employment by the Health Department of bacteriological examinations for the diagnosis of diphtheria. The appointment of Dr. William H. Park was suggested as a special inspector for this work.

This recommendation was made in view of the following considerations there detailed :

1. "The practical differentiation of diphtheria from other diseases affecting the upper air-passages is of great sanitary importance.

2. "It is admitted by all clinicians of experience in this disease that it is often impossible, either from the clinical history or the anatomical lesions or both, to make an accurate diagnosis of diphtheria. There are no constant differences which separate the simple non-contagious forms of inflammation from the diphtheritic and communicable types, and it is only in a rather small proportion of cases that an early and reliable diagnosis can be arrived at from any data obtainable. The records of the Health Department of New York City have shown this in a very striking way. In the cases of suspected diphtheria under treatment at the Willard Parker Hospital, in which the diagnoses were made by the department inspectors and confirmed by the department diagnosticians before the removal of the patients to the hospital, subsequent bacteriological examinations showed that from 30 to 50 per cent. of these cases were not diphtheria, but were cases of pseudo-diphtheria.

3. "All recent bacteriological investigations made to determine the value of such examinations for the diagnosis of diphtheria, are in accord in stating positively that reliable conclusions may be reached by this method in from twelve to twenty-four hours. These investigations include those made by Baginsky in Berlin, Martin in Paris, and Koplik and Park in New York. The results arrived at in these investigations have been confirmed by the subsequent histories of the cases

examined. In those cases in which bacteriological examinations have shown the absence of the Klebs-Loeffler bacillus, the mortality has varied from 1 to 5 per cent., and the cause of death has been usually broncho-pneumonia, and not the local disease; while in those cases in which bacteriological examinations have shown the presence of the Klebs-Loeffler bacillus, the mortality has varied from 20 to 50 per cent. Further, it has been demonstrated that in the cases in which the Klebs-Loeffler bacillus is not found, there is little danger of the transmission of the disease to others; while from the cases of true diphtheria (as shown by bacteriological examinations), even when the disease is of the mildest type, frequent and numerous instances of infection have occurred.

4. "The employment of bacteriological examinations for the diagnosis of diphtheria would have an important influence in diminishing the work of the Department and the cost of this work. Bacteriological investigations in diphtheria have shown that in most cases accurate conclusions as to the nature of the disease can be arrived at within fourteen hours. Investigations made by Dr. Park at the Willard Parker Hospital show the Department has in the past provided for the maintenance and treatment of a large number of patients having pseudo-diphtheria. This has been at a large, unnecessary cost, and the facilities of the Department for the treatment of cases of true diphtheria have been thereby limited.

"In addition to this, under the present regulations of the Department, a large number of cases of pseudo-diphtheria must be repeatedly visited by inspectors, and the rooms, clothing, etc., after convalescence, thoroughly disinfected. This is at a further large cost to the Department, and the expenditure of much valuable time.

"If the Department was prepared to avail itself at once in all cases of means for the bacteriological diagnosis of diphtheria—as this can be arrived at in so short a time—any definite action could, as a rule, be held in abeyance until a conclusion as to the nature of the disease had been reached. In those cases in which the results showed the disease was pseudo-diphtheria the Department would be at once relieved from further action.

"During the year 1891, 4,874 cases of diphtheria were reported to this Board, and so far as can be judged from the data at hand, at least $\frac{1}{3}$, and perhaps more, of these cases were not diphtheria.

5. "The resort to bacteriological examinations for the differentiation of true diphtheria from pseudo-diphtheria would constitute an important step in advance.

"The Health Department of the City of New York determined in 1892 to depend solely on bacteriological examinations for the diagnosis of Asiatic cholera. No State or municipal sanitary board has as yet officially adopted bacteriological examinations for the diagnosis of diphtheria; but in New York at least these are of far greater importance for the diagnosis of diphtheria than for the diagnosis of cholera, because of the greater prevalence and constant presence of diphtheria here. The formal recognition of this method by the Board would be received by the medical profession as an important indication of the determination of the Board to keep the work of the Department thoroughly abreast of the most recent discoveries of scientific medicine.

6. "In addition to the work in the diagnosis of diphtheria, there would naturally arise from such examinations, investigations as to the best methods to prevent the extension of the disease."

In the report just quoted, the appointment of Dr. William H. Park as Bacteriological Diagnostician and Inspector of Diphtheria was recommended, because of the investigations which had been carried on by Dr. Park during the previous year in the hospitals under the control of the Health Department, and because his special training and fitness for this position had been thoroughly demonstrated.

After some unavoidable delay, early in May, 1893, Dr. Park was appointed, in accordance with the recommendation, " Bacteriological Diagnostician and Inspector of Diphtheria."

The Board of Health, on my recommendation, then determined to make use of bacteriological examinations for the diagnosis of diphtheria, not only in all cases admitted to the hospital wards, but also in all cases of suspected diphtheria occurring in the city where the co-operation or consent of the attending physician could be obtained. This action was taken with a view to giving precision to the work of the Department in the prevention of this disease.

During the first weeks after the commencement of this work the number of cases examined weekly was comparatively small, but the number was continually increased until, during the past few months, a large proportion of all the cases of suspected diphtheria occurring in the city have been subjected to bacteriological examination.

As the scope and extent of the work increased, it was found it would be impossible for Dr. Park to make all the bacteriological examinations, and Mr. Alfred L. Beebe, Inspector of Bacteriology in this Department, was assigned to assist him.

From the beginning, those in charge of the work had little doubt of its ultimate success, but they appreciated the importance of the change that was made in the sanitary management of this disease, and did not feel assured that the physicians of this city would quickly avail themselves of the opportunities thus afforded to them.

At first, as far as possible, the Inspector of Diphtheria, or special inspectors assigned to this duty, visited physicians who reported cases of diphtheria and explained to them the purposes of the work. The Inspectors made inoculations from cases only after a request from or the consent of the attending physician had been received.

After a short trial, it was evident that a large majority of the physicians of New York would be glad to avail themselves of the assistance offered by the Department. A further step was then taken to increase the facilities for such examinations. A number of depots were established throughout the city (these now number about 40) where culture tubes and the directions required for making the inoculations could be obtained by physicians without charge.

These depots were generally established in drug stores, at convenient points, and arrangements were made for the collection of the tubes left at these depots by Department Collectors late in the afternoon of each day. For convenience and safety in transportation, small wooden boxes, containing the requisites for making a culture there, were supplied from each of the depots, i. e., a culture tube, a swab for inoculating it, and a blank for recording the name, address, etc., of the patient. Each box, with its contents, is known as "a culture outfit."

Cards giving directions for making the cultures and the addresses of the depots where tubes could be obtained were also supplied with the tubes (see below).

4

Form 20 L. 1894.Form 20 L. 1894.   2055

HEALTH DEPARTMENT—DIVISION OF PATHOLOGY, BACTERIOLOGY AND DISINFECTION, ⎱
BACTERIOLOGICAL LABORATORY,
WHITE, CENTRE, ELM AND FRANKLIN STREETS. ⎰

DIRECTIONS FOR MAKING CULTURES IN CASES OF SUSPECTED DIPHTHERIA.

The patient should be placed in a good light, and, if a child, properly held. In cases where it is possible to get a good view of the throat, depress the tongue and rub the cotton swab gently, but freely, against any visible exudate. In other cases, including those in which the exudate is confined to the larynx, avoiding the tongue, pass the swab far back, and rub it freely against the mucous membrane of the pharynx and tonsils. Without laying the swab down, withdraw the cotton plug from the culture tube, insert the swab, and rub that portion of it which has touched the exudate gently but thoroughly back and forth all over the surface of the blood serum. Do not push the swab into the blood serum, nor break the surface in any way. Replace the swab in its own tube, plug both tubes, put them in the box, and return the culture outfit at once to the station from which it was obtained.

A report will be forwarded the following morning by mail, or can be obtained by telephone, after 12 noon.

Culture outfits can be obtained from the following stations free of cost :

East side—
No. 712 Tremont avenue..Eichwort
One Hundred and Thirty-eighth street and Third avenue...........................Fraser
One Hundred and Twenty-fifth street and Madison avenue.........................Marsh
One Hundred and Sixteenth street and Third avenue............................Engelhardt
One Hundred and Fifteenth street and First avenue..............................New
One Hundred and Tenth street and Madison avenue...............................Barnes
One Hundred and Fifth street and Third avenue ....Aaronstam
Eighty-sixth street and Park avenue.......................................Falkenrecht
Sixty-seventh street and Third avenue.....................................Hoykendorff
Forty-fifth street and Third avenue ....Goetting
Forty-second street and Park avenue.....................................Schoonmaker
Forty-first street and Park avenue....................................Van Horn & Ellison
Twenty-ninth street and Fourth avenue..Bagoe
Twelfth street and Second avenue..Proben
Eleventh street and Avenue A ....Montesser
Spring street and Bowery ....Minor

West side—
One Hundred and Thirty-fifth street and Seventh avenue ....Breen
One Hundred and Twenty-fifth street and Eighth avenue ....Spear
One Hundred and Twenty-second street and Seventh avenue.................Heinemann
Ninety-eighth street and Columbus avenue ....Rosenson
Ninety-third street and Columbus avenue.......................................Dorn
Seventy-second street and Boulevard..Kerley
Seventy-second street and Columbus avenue..................................Cassabeer
No. 411 West Fifty-ninth street...Dougherty
Forty-sixth street and Fifth avenue..................................Bartlett & Liell
Thirty-sixth street and Ninth avenue...Rupp
Twenty-ninth street and Fifth avenue ....Frazer
Twenty-second street and Ninth avenue ....Smith

West side—

 No. 157 Eighth avenue...Lins
 No. 148 Eighth avenue...Utley
 Twelfth street and Sixth avenue..Ridgeway
 Eighth street and Sixth avenue...Bigelow
 No. 283 Bleecker street...McCord
 No. 172 Varick street...Jennsen

Form of blank with each "Culture Outfit" :

21 L. 1894.   ☞ Return swab and both tubes.   2058

DIPHTHERIA.

Name of Maker of Culture
Date   Time
Name of Patient   Age
Address
Att. Phys.   Address
Duration of Disease
How Contracted
Can Case be Isolated ?
Location of Membrane
Was Inoculation Satisfactory ?
Clinical Diagnosis

☞ Return swab and both tubes.

The diagnosticians, and later the Medical Inspectors of the Department, were supplied with leather pocket cases containing a number of culture tubes and swabs, and were given instructions regarding the methods of making the inoculations. These arrangements being completed, the following circular was delivered, by special messengers, at the office of every physician in this city :

HEALTH DEPARTMENT,   }
NEW YORK, July, 1893.   {

CIRCULAR OF INFORMATION CONCERNING THE USE OF BACTERIAL CULTURES FOR THE DIAGNOSIS OF DIPHTHERIA.

Recent bacterial investigations have shown that a considerable proportion of the cases of pseudo-membranous and exudative inflammations of the throat and upper air passages, commonly considered as diphtheria, and having the anatomical appearances found in diphtheria, are not true diphtheria. These cases may be called pseudo or false diphtheria.

It has also been shown that a considerable number of cases which are apparently false diphtheria prove on bacterial examination to be true diphtheria. While in true diphtheria the mortality is very high and the danger of transmission to others is great, in false diphtheria the mortality is low and the danger of infection slight. The differential diagnosis between true and false diphtheria can be made by bacteriological examination within fourteen hours, while without this the differentiation is difficult or impossible.

The Health Department is now prepared to make use of bacterial cultures for diagnosis in all cases of suspected diphtheria occurring in the city, and desires that in every case either the physicians should themselves make the inoculations, or should authorize an Inspector to make them. They should be made in every suspicious case at the earliest possible moment, for during convalescence the specific organisms often disappear from the throat and the full benefit of a positive diagnosis is not obtained unless it is made early in the disease.

The inoculations are made by gently rubbing a cotton swab against the throat, and then drawing it over the surface of the culture-medium. When the physician desires to himself make the culture (and this is usually the better plan, for it can be done earlier and is more agreeable to the family), he can obtain, free of cost, a culture-tube and swab, and the simple directions necessary for their use, at any one of the druggists whose addresses are given below. After the inoculation the tubes are to be returned at once to the druggist from whom they were obtained. The tubes will be collected by the Department every evening.

In cases where an inoculation has not been made by the attending physician, the Medical Inspector will make one, unless for some reason the physician requests that none be made when he notifies the Department of the case.

The diagnosis will be ready by noon of the following day. The attending physician can obtain it immediately by telephoning to the laboratory, or when this is not done he will be notified by mail. Cases which prove to be false diphtheria will not be visited by the Health Department Inspectors. Cases, on the other hand, which prove to be true diphtheria, will be subjected to the usual rules and regulations covering contagious diseases.

The materials required for making inoculations can be obtained from the following druggists free of cost:

All communications on this subject should be addressed to Dr. Hermann M. Biggs, Chief Inspector, Division of Pathology, Bacteriology and Disinfection, No. 42 Bleecker street (Telephone " 1191 Spring ").

By order of the Board of Health,

CHARLES G. WILSON, President.

EMMONS CLARK, Secretary.

As soon as it was possible to still further enlarge the work, a new investigation was instituted. This was to determine by the bacteriological examination of secondary cultures made from the throats of convalescent cases of diphtheria, how long the bacilli of diphtheria persist during convalescence.

After a number of examinations had been made sufficient to draw accurate conclusions, the following circular was printed, and ordered to be sent to physicians with the report of the result of the bacteriological examination of the first culture. In it the important announcement is made that in the future no case will be considered free of the contagion of diphtheria until this fact has been established by culture test.

Form 31 L.

HEALTH DEPARTMENT, No. 301 MOTT STREET,
DIVISION OF PATHOLOGY, BACTERIOLOGY AND DISINFECTION,
No. 42 BLEECKER STREET (Telephone, 1191 Spring),
NEW YORK,...............189..)

To Dr.. ...

SIR -- During the last few months a series of investigations have been made in the bacteriological laboratory of the Health Department to determine how long the Loeffler bacilli remain in the throat in cases of diphtheria after the disappearance of all false membrane. The results obtained are extremely significant, and have caused the Department to establish new regulations regarding the discharge from observation of patients who have suffered from diphtheria, and regarding the time of disinfection of the premises.

During the past three months 405 cases of true diphtheria have been subjected to repeated bacteriological examinations performed at short intervals during the course of the disease and during convalescence. In all of these cases cultures were made at the beginning of the disease, again after the lapse of three or four days, and finally at short periods after the complete disappearance of the false membrane, until the throat was found to be free from the diphtheria bacillus. In 245 of these 405 cases the diphtheria bacilli disappeared within three days after the complete separation of the false membrane ; in 160 cases the diphtheria bacilli persisted for a longer time, namely : in 103 cases for seven days, in 34 cases for twelve days, in 16 cases for fifteen days, in 4 cases for three weeks and in 3 cases for five weeks after the time when the exudation had completely disappeared from the upper air passages. In many of these cases the patients were apparently well many days before the infectious agent had disappeared from the throat. These results show that in a considerable proportion of cases persons who have had diphtheria continue to carry the germs of the disease in their throats for many days after all signs and symptoms of the disease have disappeared. No doubt the disease is largely disseminated by these persons who are apparently well, and who mingle with others while their throat secretions still contain the diphtheria bacilli.

These experiments have led the Health Department to adopt the rule, that no person who has suffered from diphtheria shall be considered free from contagion until it has been shown, by a bacteriological examination, made after the disappearance of the membrane from the throat, that the throat secretions no longer contain the diphtheria bacilli, and until such examinations have shown such absence all cases in boarding houses, hotels and tenement houses must remain isolated and under observation. Disinfection of the premises there will not be performed by the Department until examination has shown the absence of the diphtheria bacilli.

Secondary cultures, as well as primary cultures, may be made by the attending physician, if he so desires ; otherwise they will be made by the inspector of the district in which the case occurs. This applies only to cases occurring in boarding houses, hotels and tenement houses—not to those in private houses.

It has been noticed that, occasionally, when culture tubes are inoculated immediately after irrigation of the throat with antiseptic solutions, the cultures do not show any Loeffler bacilli, although subsequent examinations may demonstrate their presence. This observation should be noted in making inoculations.

Very respectfully,

HERMANN M. BIGGS, M. D.,
Chief Inspector of Pathology, Bacteriology and Disinfection.

Approved by the Board of Health,

CHARLES G. WILSON, President.
EMMONS CLARK, Secretary.

Blank to be Filled Out and Returned with Secondary Cultures.

26 L. 1894. ☞Return swab and both tubes. 2057

DIPHTHERIA.—Later Cultures.

Number of Culture, 2d, 3d, 4th, 5th, 6th, 7th, 8th.
Date   Inspector or Physician
Name of Patient   Laboratory Number
Address
Duration of Disease
Is the place ready for disinfection if the culture is found free from diphtheria bacilli ?

During the first few months, in order to test the results of the examinations and to make the liability to error as slight as possible, the following plan was adopted :

All cases which yielded no diphtheria bacilli were turned over to Special Inspectors, who made, if possible, in every case a second culture, and followed up the patient for some time after recovery.

From the information thus secured, the Bacteriologists of the Department were able to decide more and more surely how far they could base an absolute diagnosis on the examination of a culture.

In the circular given above, the Board of Health announced that cases which proved on bacteriological examination to be false diphtheria would not be kept under the observation of the Department. Some physicians who heartily approved of the work of the Department in its treatment of diphtheria, believed that in this step it had proceeded too far, and that the false cases, though less contagious than the true, were yet sufficiently so to render isolation and supervision necessary. From a large experience, the Board of Health believed these cases were so rarely serious in their results and were so little, if at all, contagious, that visits from Department Inspectors were unnecessary. Nevertheless, before issuing the circular, 150 consecutive cases were investigated, all sources of contagion sought for, and the patients kept under observation for two weeks after convalescence. In none of these was isolation or disinfection required. The evidence obtained so completely confirmed the previous experience that the Board of Health felt justified in concluding it was unnecessary to exercise any sanitary supervision over cases of false diphtheria. Those who believe they have met with cases of false diphtheria which have been the cause of severe or fatal illness in others, have probably either mistaken the nature of the first case, or have been dealing with some other infectious disease (such as scarlet fever), in which the inflammation of the throat is merely a secondary lesion.

In order to make the possibility of error in the routine work as small as possible, for some months the following circular has been mailed to physicians with every report :

HEALTH DEPARTMENT,
DIVISION OF PATHOLOGY, BACTERIOLOGY AND DISINFECTION,
NO. 42 BLEECKER STREET,
NEW YORK, February 20, 1894.

To Physicians :

It is the earnest desire of the Health Department that the service in the bacteriological diagnosis of diphtheria be made as perfect as possible and as useful to physicians as it can be made. When cultures are left at any of the depots before 4 P. M., it is the aim to return in every case a report of the bacteriological diagnosis on the following day. Reports are mailed before one o'clock, and should be delivered to the physician before the last mail of the day. Earlier reports can be obtained by applying to the Laboratory by telephone after 12 M.

When the bacteriological diagnosis does not harmonize with the clinical facts and the history, as shown by antecedent or subsequent cases of diphtheria, and where there are any defects or reasons for complaint regarding the service in any respect, physicians are earnestly requested to report these promptly to the Chief Inspector, Dr. H. M. Biggs, No. 42 Bleecker street. Knowledge of defects in the service can only reach the Department through such reports, and the service can only thus be improved and perfected.

9

Physicians are requested to read carefully the accompanying circulars describing the character of the work and the method of procedure, and to follow exactly the instruction given. Thus uniformity in method and accuracy in results will be insured.

HERMANN M. BIGGS, M. D.,
Chief Inspector of Pathology, Bacteriology and Disinfection.

Depending on the results obtained from the examination of primary cultures, one of the following blanks is filled out and mailed to the attending physician before 12 M. of the day following that on which the culture was made :

22 L. 1894. Laboratory 2056

HEALTH DEPARTMENT,
DIVISION OF PATHOLOGY, BACTERIOLOGY AND DISINFECTION,
BACTERIOLOGICAL LABORATORY, CENTRE, WHITE, ELM AND FRANKLIN STREETS,
NEW YORK,................ ...189..

Dr............................. ....

DEAR SIR—The examination of the culture made by inoculating the tube with the exudation from the throat of......................,.......on..................................... shows the presence of the diphtheria bacilli.

The case is therefore one of true diphtheria.

.....................................Chief Inspector.

....Inspector of Diphtheria.

24 Form L.

HEALTH DEPARTMENT,
DIVISION OF PATHOLOGY, BACTERIOLOGY AND DISINFECTION,
BACTERIOLOGICAL LABORATORY, No. 42 BLEECKER STREET,
NEW YORK,....................189..

Dr..................................... .....

DEAR SIR—The examination of the cultures made by inoculating the tube with the exudation from the throat of.....................................on...................................... does not show the presence of any diphtheria bacilli.

The case is therefore not true diphtheria,* but pseudo or false diphtheria, and no further cognizance will be taken of it by the Department unless by the special request of the physician in attendance.

.....................................Chief Inspector.

....Inspector of Diphtheria.

32 Form L.

HEALTH DEPARTMENT,
DIVISION OF PATHOLOGY, BACTERIOLOGY AND DISINFECTION,
BACTERIOLOGICAL LABORATORY, No. 42 BLEECKER STREET,
NEW YORK,....................189..

Dr..................................... ....

DEAR SIR—The examination of the cultures made by inoculating the tube with the exudation from the throat of.....................................on.............................. does not admit of an exact bacteriological diagnosis, for the following reasons :

* This conclusion is based on the supposition that the directions have been carefully followed and that the inoculation was made before the commencement of convalescence. After convalescence is established the bacilli often disappear from the exudate.

A. The inoculation was made at so late a period in the disease that it is possible that the diphtheria bacilli, though now absent, were at an earlier time present.

B. The growth on the culture media was so scanty that it is probable that the inoculation was not properly made, or that some antiseptic had been applied to the throat shortly before obtaining the material for inoculating the tube.

C. The culture media was contaminated.

D. The serum in the tube was too dry to permit of the growth of the diphtheria bacilli.

a. Another culture is requested.

b. The case will be treated as one of diphtheria.

c. The case will be treated as one of false diphtheria unless the physician in charge of the case requests otherwise.

....Chief Inspector.

....Inspector of Diphtheria.

After the examination of each secondary culture, and depending on the result of the examination, one of the following blanks is filled out and forwarded to the attending physician and to the Chief Inspector of Disinfection :

27 L. 1894.   Laboratory No.........   2060

HEALTH DEPARTMENT,
DIVISION OF PATHOLOGY, BACTERIOLOGY AND DISINFECTION,
BACTERIOLOGICAL LABORATORY, CENTRE, WHITE, ELM AND FRANKLIN STREETS,
NEW YORK,....................189..

Dr...................... ....

DEAR SIR—The examination of the culture made by inoculating the tube from the throat of
....on..................... ....
shows the presence of the diphtheria bacilli.

The case is therefore not yet ready for disinfection, but needs a further culture.

....Chief Inspector.

....Inspector of Diphtheria.

28 L. 1894.   Laboratory No.........   2061

HEALTH DEPARTMENT,
DIVISION OF PATHOLOGY, BACTERIOLOGY AND DISINFECTION,
BATERIOLOGICAL LABORATORY, CENTRE, WHITE, ELM AND FRANKLIN STREETS,
NEW YORK, ...189..

Dr...

DEAR SIR—The examination of the culture made by inoculating the tube from the throat of
....on..................... ....
does not show the presence of any diphtheria bacilli.

The case is therefore ready for disinfection, if the other circumstances allow.

....Chief Inspector.

....Inspector of Diphtheria.

In the beginning of this work, some physicians familiar with bacteriological work feared it was unwise to trust the inoculation of the culture tubes to physicians unskilled in bacteriological methods. The Department has found, however, that physicians may, as a rule, be relied on to carefully follow the simple directions given for making inoculations of culture tubes, and that the diagnosis based on the results obtained from the bacteriological examinations of such tubes can be safely accepted.

A communication was forwarded to the Board of Health in November, 1893, recommending the adoption of an amendment to the Sanitary Code which should include so-called "membranous croup" with the contagious diseases, concerning which the Department requires reports from physicians. This recommendation was based on the results of the bacteriological examinations of a considerable number of cases of croup, which showed that more than 80 per cent. of them were really cases of laryngeal diphtheria.

The detailed results of the work for the first year, both as to the bacteriological examination of cases of suspected diphtheria and the experimental work on questions allied to this, are contained in the appended report from the Bacteriological Laboratory, by Dr. William H. Park, Bacteriological Diagnostician and Inspector of Diphtheria, and Mr. Alfred L. Beebe, Inspector of Bacteriology, by whom the work has been performed.

The question is naturally and properly asked, as to what influence this work has had on the prevalence of diphtheria in this city? In reply to this it can only be said that there has been a very large increase in the number of cases of diphtheria occurring during the last year in many of the large cities of the world, and New York has suffered from this semi-epidemic influence, but to a much less extent than some other cities. The number of cases reported weekly had begun to increase before the initiation of this work, and this increase has continued notwithstanding it. The total number of cases reported during the last year has been considerably greater than during the previous year, but the number of cases, apparently occurring in the city, has been unquestionably increased by the more universal reporting of cases by physicians. It is, of course, impossible to say how much greater the real increase of cases would have been without the work which has been carried on by the Department. The inability of the Department to completely control the spread of the disease will be readily understood by reference to the description of the methods of dissemination of the disease contained in the detailed report from the Bacteriological Laboratory.

It may be said in conclusion that the success of this new departure of the Health Department of New York City has far exceeded all anticipation. The Board of Health was the first sanitary Board in the world to officially adopt and provide for the making of such bacteriological examinations, and the course of the Board in this matter has been carefully watched by the sanitary authorities in various parts of the world. Constant inquiries have been made as to the conduct of the work and many requests for circulars and for information as to the manner in which the work is carried on have been received. Numerous representatives of other health departments have been instructed in the Bacteriological Laboratory, in the methods employed, and the plan of work, as devised by this Department, has been adopted, without modification, by the Health authorities of many other cities.

Respectfully submitted,

HERMANN M. BIGGS,
Pathologist, and Director of the Bacteriological Laboratory.

A Report on the Bacteriological Examination of 5,611 Cases of Suspected Diphtheria, with the Results of Other Investigations on the Diphtheria and the Pseudo-Diphtheria Bacillus.

By William Hallock Park, M. D., Bacteriological Diagnostician and Inspector of Diphtheria, and Alfred L. Beebe, Ph. B., Inspector of Bacteriology, to Herman M. Biggs, M. D., Pathologist and Director of the Bacteriological Laboratory.

From May 4, 1893, to May 4, 1894, there were 5,611 cases of suspected diphtheria subjected to bacteriological examination. In 3,255 of these the Loeffler bacilli (the bacilli of true diphtheria) were found to be present, and these cases were thus proven to be true diphtheria. In 1,540 no diphtheria bacilli were present in the cultures; and as these had been carefully made at an early period of the disease, the cases from which they were taken may be considered as proven not to have been true diphtheria. In 816 cases, although no diphtheria bacilli were found in the cultures, yet, for various reasons (either because they were made after the fourth day of the disease, or the exudate was imperfectly obtained from the throat or the culture media had become contaminated or were too dry) the cases from which the cultures were obtained were considered to be of a doubtful nature, as far as the bacteriological examination was concerned, although they were probably not diphtheria.

Thus we find in 5,611 cases of suspected diphtheria that about 58 per cent. were proven to be true diphtheria, 27 per cent. to be false or pseudo-diphtheria, and 15 per cent. to be of a somewhat doubtful character. It would probably be just to consider that 60 per cent. were true and 40 per cent. were false diphtheria.

SEX, AGE AND MORTALITY IN THE CASES OF TRUE DIPHTHERIA.

In a large percentage of the cases the sex was given, and in these there were 54 per cent. females and 46 per cent. males, a fairly even division. The statistics reveal some interesting facts as to the influence of age on the occurrence of true diphtheria, as well as on the mortality of the disease. The ages of persons attacked ranged between three weeks and seventy years. The number of cases increased with each twelve months of life up to the fourth year and then gradually diminished. The mortality was highest in the first two years of life and then steadily diminished until adult life was reached, when it again slowly increased. The ages and mortality were determined in 1,625 cases, and were as follows :

Age.	Number of Cases.	Mortality.	Age.	Number of Cases.	Number of Cases per Year, Average.	Mortality.
First 12 months......	24		7th to 10th year........	292	97+	15 per cent.
Second "	109		10th to 15th year........	117	23+	5 "
Third "	233	45 per cent.	15th to 20th year........	20	4	
Fourth "	258		20th to 30th year........	41	4+	20 "
Fifth "	192		30th to 50th year........	13	13 to 20	
Sixth "	163	33 "				
Seventh "	163		Total mortality in all cases............			27 per cent.

Scarlet fever was associated with diphtheria in about five of every thousand cases. Exact figures cannot be given.

The 5 deaths occurring in uncomplicated pseudo-diphtheria in children under five years of age were all in cases in which the larynx was affected, and in 3, more or less broncho-pneumonia developed as a complication.

AGE AND MORTALITY IN FALSE OR PSEUDO-DIPHTHERIA.

It has been the general rule of the Department to take no further cognizance of cases of false diphtheria after the culture has demonstrated the absence of the diphtheria bacilli.

In order, however, to compare the mortality and the communicability of false diphtheria with that of true diphtheria, 450 cases of the false were carefully investigated by sanitary inspectors detailed for this work. These cases comprised 300 occurring in the Fall months and 150 occurring in the following Spring. The cases were taken in consecutive order, and are believed to be average cases.

Age.	Number of Cases.	Number of Deaths.	Mortality.	Age.	Number of Cases.	Average per Year.	Number of Deaths.	Mortality.
First 12 months	2	0		7th to 10th year.	63	21	..	0
Second "	17	5*		10th to 15th year.	63	12+	..	0
Third "	47	0	7 per cent.	15th to 20th year.	44	9—	..	0
Fourth "	36	2†		20th to 30th year.	63	6+	1	
Fifth "	30	2‡		30th to 50th year.	17	1—	..	2⅔ per cent.
Sixth "	34	0	2 per cent.	Over 50 years ...	2	..	1	
Seventh "	32	0						

* Two deaths due to scarlet fever.   † One death due to scarlet fever.   ‡ One death due to scarlet fever.

In the 450 cases investigated there were 11 deaths, or about 2½ per cent. mortality. Of the 450 cases, 42 were complicated by scarlet fever, and of these 42, 4 died. In six of the 450 cases, measles occurred as a complication, and these all recovered. Of the 2 deaths which occurred among the adults, 1 was of a man of 70 years, who was suffering from a serious valvular lesion of the heart, and the other was of a young adult female,* who died of septicæmia.

TRUE AND PSEUDO-DIPHTHERIA OF THE LARYNX.

(Membranous Croup.)

The statistics gathered of the location of the disease in the true and false cases are of special interest. There were 286 of the cases examined in which the disease was entirely or chiefly confined to the larynx or bronchi, and of these, 283 were in children and 3 in adults. In the cultures

---

* NOTE.—The history, in brief, of the second case was as follows: Three weeks before death the disease began with a swelling of 1 tonsil and its surrounding tissues. A week later the tonsil was incised, but no pus obtained, and about the incision a dirty brown pseudo-membrane formed. Later, the tonsil and its surrounding tissue became necrotic and sloughed off ; then the ulceration extended to the pharynx and the other tonsil, and was still progressing, when the patient died of sepsis and exhaustion.

of 229 of the 286, characteristic Loeffler bacilli were found, and the cases were thus proven to be true diphtheria. Of the 229 cases in which the Loeffler bacilli were found, 167 showed no pseudo-membrane or exudate above larnyx, while in the remaining 62, although the larnyx was mainly involved, there was also some membrane or exudate present on the tonsils or in the pharynx. In 57 out of the 286 examined, no diphtheria bacilli were found, but in 17 of these the cultures were unsatisfactory. Excluding the 17 doubtful cases, there were 40 cases of pseudo-diphtheria in which the diphtheria bacilli were certainly absent. The disease was confined to the larynx or bronchi in 27 out of the 40, while more or less exudate or membrane was present on the tonsils or in the pharynx in 13.

Table of Results of Examinations of Cases of " Membranous Croup."

	Diphtheria Bacilli Found.	Diphtheria Bacilli Not Found.
Cases in which the exudate was confined to the larynx or bronchi..	167	27
Cases in which the exudate was chiefly confined to the larynx or bronchi, but other parts somewhat involved..............	62	13
Cases in which satisfactory cultures were not obtained...................................		17
Total cases examined..		286
Diphtheria............		229
Pseudo-diphtheria...		40
Doubtful...		17

We find, therefore, that of the cases of acute laryngitis in children which have been subjected to bacteriological examination in the laboratory of the Health Department during the past twelve months, about 80 per cent. have proved to be undoubtedly cases of diphtheria, and of the remaining 20 per cent. only 14 per cent. were certainly not diphtheritic.

Not only have the bacteriological examinations shown that a large proportion of the cases of acute croupous laryngitis in children (commonly designated by the name membranous croup) are diphtheria, but the Department Inspectors have frequently found that these cases were apparently the cause of characteristic pharyngeal diphtheria in others.

The comparatively small number of laryngeal cases examined is partially due to the fact that membranous croup has not been considered a contagious disease, and reports of such cases have not been required by the Health Department ; and partially to the custom of Department Inspectors to not make cultures in cases which have been intubated, or which seem so sick that the family may think injury has been done by inserting the swab in the throat. The cases in which no cultures are made are treated as cases of true diphtheria.

An amendment to the Sanitary Code was adopted by the Board of Health on June 6, 1894, by virtue of which membranous croup is regarded as laryngeal diphtheria, and hereafter physicians will be required to report such cases to the Health Department.

NOTE--Many experienced physicians still find difficulty in believing that cases in which the exudate or pseudo-membrane is entirely absent from the pharynx and tonsils are those of true diphtheria. It is also often difficult to persuade parents that such cases are diphtheria, as for instance, a child, aged five, subject to attacks of bronchitis and slight laryngitis, developed a croupy cough. For diagnostic purposes, a culture was made and the diphtheria bacilli were found to be present. It was with the greatest difficulty that the parents could be made to consider the case a serious one and to quarantine the child. Under suitable treatment, on the fifth day the child seemed nearly recovered, and now the parents became sure it was not a case of diphtheria, stopped all precautions, allowed the child to go out, etc. A relapse followed, the laryngeal symptoms increased, and the child died in thirty-eight hours, of asphyxia, intubation being refused.

THE RELATION BETWEEN THE LENGTH OF THE BACILLUS AND ITS VIRULENCE.

Some investigators have believed the degree of virulence possessed by the diphtheria bacilli could, to a certain extent, be judged by their length. The longest bacilli were supposed to be the most virulent, those of medium length less so, and the shortest, little if at all virulent. By observing this characteristic it was thought cultures might become helpful in prognosis. Very careful notes have been made on this point in the examination of the bacteria from the original serum tubes in 1,613 cases.

The results of the examinations are shown in the following table :

	NUMBER OF CASES.	MORTALITY.
Bacilli of average size found in....................................	1,398	26 per cent.
Bacilli longer than average in	82	27 "
Bacilli shorter than average in....................................	67	35 "
Bacilli short, not characteristic in shape and evenly stained, of which many were pseudo-diphtheria bacilli.......................	66	12 "
Number of cases examined..	1,613	

The results obtained from this examination of 1,613 cultures therefore indicate that in New York the great majority of cases of diphtheria yield in cultures bacilli of medium size, which are characteristic in shape and manner of staining. In a moderate number of cases, the bacilli found are much longer, and in about an equal number they are much shorter. Both the clinical histories and the animal experiments show that whenever in their shape and in the way in which they take the staining fluid the bacilli are characteristic, no information as to their virulence, either in men or animals, can be gathered from their length. Those bacilli, on the other hand, which are short and stain uniformly with methyl blue, usually prove to be of the pseudo-diphtheria type, and have no virulence in animals.

THE BACTERIOLOGY OF DIPHTHERIA.

So many inquiries have been sent to the Department regarding the methods employed for the general bacteriological examinations of suspected cases of diphtheria, that it has been thought desirable to include in this report a condensed account of the new facts which have been brought out in the various bacteriological investigations made on this subject, together with a description of the characteristics of the diphtheria bacilli which must be known in order to make bacterio logical examinations for diagnostic purposes.

It is hoped that with these additions this report may be of greater practical assistance to many who have begun or are about to begin similar work.

Successive Investigations Showing the Specific Causal Relation of the Diphtheria Bacillus of Klebs and Loeffler to Diphtheria.

In the year 1883, bacilli which were very peculiar and striking in appearance were shown by Klebs (1) to be of constant occurrence in the pseudo-membranes from the throats of those dying of true epidemic diphtheria. One year later, Loeffler (2) published the results of a very thorough and extensive series of investigations on this subject. He found the bacillus described by Klebs in most but not all cases of throat inflammations which had been diagnosticated as diphtheria. He separated these bacilli from the other bacteria present and obtained them in pure culture. When he inoculated these bacilli upon the abraded mucous membrane of susceptible animals, pseudo-membranes were produced, and frequently death followed. If a certain amount of a bouillon culture was injected subcutaneously into guinea pigs, death was caused with characteristic lesions. Loeffler's failure to find the bacilli in every case examined is now explained by the fact that certain varieties of pseudo-membranous inflammation not due to the diphtheria bacillus, such as occur especially in scarlet fever, were then wrongly considered to be true diphtheria.

In 1887 (3) further studies by Loeffler added to the proof of the dependence of diphtheria on the diphtheria bacilli. In 1888 D'Espiné found the bacilli in 14 cases of characteristic diphtheria, and proves them to be absent in 24 cases of mild sore throats which, clinically, were believed not to be cases of diphtheria. In the same year, the first portion of the results of the very important investigations of Roux (4) and Yersin was published, and the dependence of diphtheria on the diphtheria bacilli may be considered to have been established. Roux and Yersin found the diphtheria bacilli were present in all characteristic cases of diphtheria, and that these bacilli possessed the cultural and pathogenic qualities of those described by Loeffler. They found, too, when the bacilli were inoculated upon the healthy mucous membrane of the trachea of the rabbit, no result followed ; but, if the inoculation was made on the abraded membrane, phenomena occurred, which strikingly resembled those present in membranous laryngitis in man, i. e., congestion of the mucous membrane, followed by the formation of a pseudo-membrane, œdematous swelling of the tissues and of the glands of the neck, dyspnœa, stridulous breathing and asphyxia. Injection of cultures beneath the skin of rabbits and guinea pigs in sufficient quantity caused their death in from thirty-six hours to five days, the period varying in ratio to the susceptibility of the animal, and the number and violence of the bacteria introduced. The same result followed the injections of filtered cultures, showing the products formed by the growth of the bacilli were, by themselves, capable of causing the general lesions.

Roux and Yersin were also able to produce in animals characteristic diphtheria paralysis. They produced this in many cases where the inoculated animals did not succumb to a too rapid intoxication. Paralysis commenced in a pigeon three weeks after the inoculation of the pharynx, and after all membrane had disappeared and the animal seemed to have completely recovered.

In rabbits the paralysis usually commenced in the posterior extremities and then gradually extended to the whole body, causing death by paralysis of the heart or respiration. In rare instances, the muscles of the neck or of the larynx were first paralyzed, and thus characteristic symptoms were caused. The authors conclude, " the occurrence of these paralyses, following the introduction of the bacilli of Klebs and Loeffler, completes the resemblance of the experimental disease to the natural malady, and establishes with certainty the specific rule of this bacillus."

Finally, the microscopic changes in the internal organs of animals dying of experimental diphtheria produced by the bacilli have been shown by Welch and Flexner (5), and by Babes (6) and others to be essentially the same as those produced by diphtheria in man, and thus a still further proof is afforded of the specific role of this bacillus.

The results of the various observations detailed above have since been confirmed by a great number of combined clinical and bacteriological investigations, so that all who have studied the bacteriology of diphtheria would now agree with the following statement made by Welch (7) in an address on diphtheria : " All the conditions have been fulfilled for diphtheria which are necessary to the most rigid proof of the dependence of an infective disease upon a given micro-organism, viz., the constant presence of this organism in the lesions of the disease, the isolation of the organism in pure culture, the reproduction of the disease by inoculations of pure cultures, and similar distribution of the organism in the experimental and in the natural disease. In view of these facts, we must agree with Prudden (8) that we are now justified in saying that the name diphtheria, or at least primary diphtheria, should be applied, and exclusively applied, to that acute infectious disease usually associated with pseudo-membranous affection of the mucous membrane which is primarily caused by the bacillus called the bacillus diphtheriæ of Loeffler."

Pseudo or False Diphtheria.

Under this general title are included all cases of pseudo-membranous or exudative inflammation of the mucous membranes in which the diphtheria bacillus is absent.

The thorough consideration of the bacteriology of this form of inflammation is to be reserved for a later report, but it is necessary to touch on a few points here.

Since Loeffler (2), in 1889, first described a class of pseudo-membranous inflammations of the throat in which the diphtheria bacilli were absent and cocci present, it has been established that a certain proportion of the inflammations of the respiratory mucous membranes, which closely resemble the less characteristic cases of diphtheria, are not due to the diphtheria bacilli, but to cocci, especially to streptococci.

It has been found that streptococci are commonly present in the throats of healthy persons, or at least in the throats of persons living in large cities, and that other forms of cocci, especially the pneumo-cocci, and staphylococci are apt to be associated with them. These germs seem to live in the throat without creating any disturbance there, so long as the mucous membranes are healthy, but under certain conditions, as when the mucous membrane has been made vulnerable by exposure to cold or other deleterious influences, or by the poison of scarlet fever, measles or some other disease, the streptococci, alone or associated with other cocci, are able to attack the mucous membrane and to cause an inflammation. This may be of any degree of intensity, from a simple

2

inflammatory hyperania to an inflammation with the extensive production of pseudo-membrane or with ulceration. Such inflammations when associated with the formation of a pseudo-membrane are known as pseudo-diphtheria. The exudate or pseudo-membrane in pseudo-diphtheria is usually confined to the tonsils, but other parts, such as the larynx, pharynx and nostrils, may be invaded.

It has been found that the percentage of mortality in these cases is far less than in diphtheria, and that the disease is seldom, if ever, communicated to others.

The Proportion of Cases of Suspected Diphtheria which upon Examination Prove to be True Diphtheria.

As soon as careful investigation had demonstrated it was possible, with proper precautions, to separate by bacteriological examination the cases of the true from the cases of the false diphtheria, large numbers of cases suspected to be diphtheria were examined bacteriologically. The reports from hospitals in which all cases of suspected diphtheria were examined are of special interest as showing the proportion of cases of true to false diphtheria. The results from these hospitals are all the more valuable because the cases came from all parts of the various cities in which the respective hospitals were located, and hence special local conditions were not likely to greatly influence the general results obtained. Thus, Baginsky (9), in Berlin, found the diphtheria bacilli in 120 out of 154 suspected cases; Martin (10), in Paris, in 126 out of 200; Park (11), in New York, in 127 out of 244; Janson (12), in Switzerland, in 63 out of 100, and Morse (13), in Boston, in 239 out of 400. Thus, from 20 to 50 per cent. of the cases sent to diphtheria hospitals did not have diphtheria.

If we examine the reports of examinations made under some special conditions, as during an outbreak of some contagious disease in a hospital for children, we find the results may differ in a striking manner.

Thus, in 1889, Prudden (14) made bacteriological examinations of 24 fatal cases of pseudo-membranous inflammation of the tonsils, pharynx and larynx. In none of these were the Loeffler bacilli found to be present. These cases occurred in 2 hospitals for children in New York, in which both scarlet fever and measles were at the time prevalent. During the past year we have examined the exudate from 46 fatal cases of suspected diphtheria occurring in these same institutions and found the bacilli present in 44 of them.

If scarlet fever and measles (but not true diphtheria) were prevailing in an institution, it is evident the bacilli would be absent from the pseudo-membranes occasionally occurring in the throat as a complication of these diseases.

The Mortality in True Diphtheria and in Pseudo-Diphtheria.

All observers have found the mortality far higher in those cases in which the diphtheria bacilli were present than in those in which they were absent. In true diphtheria the mortality has been found to vary from 25 to 70 per cent., while in pseudo-diphtheria it varies from 0 per cent. to 20 per cent.

The death rate in cases of pseudo-diphtheria occurring in hospitals averages far higher than the death rate outside of such institutions. The reason for this is chiefly to be found in the fact that it is mainly the graver cases, especially those suffering from laryngeal obstruction, which are removed to the hospitals.

LABORATORY TECHNIQUE.

Collection of the Blood Serum and its Preparation for Use in Cultures.

A covered glass jar, which has been thoroughly cleansed with hot water, is taken to the slaughter-house and filled with freshly shed blood from a calf or sheep. The blood is received directly in the jar as it spurts from the cut in the throat of the animal. After wiping the edge of the jar, it is covered with the lid and set aside where it may stand quietly until the blood has thoroughly clotted. The jar is then carried to the laboratory and placed in an ice chest. If the jar containing the blood is carried about before the latter has clotted, very imperfect separation of the serum will take place. It is well to inspect the blood in the jar after it has been standing a few hours, and if the clot is found adhering to the sides, to separate it by a rod. The blood is allowed to remain twenty-four hours on the ice, and then the serum which surrounds the clot is siphoned off by a rubber tube and mixed with one-third its quantity of nutrient beef broth, to which 1 per cent. glucose has been added. This constitutes the Loeffler blood serum mixture. The broth used to mix with the serum is prepared as follows: One pound of finely chopped lean beef is allowed to soak in one liter of water in a cool place for at least twelve hours. The meat and fluid are now dumped into a cheese-cloth or towel, and the fluid squeezed out. To this solution 1 per cent. of peptone, 1 per cent. of glucose and ½ per cent. of common salt are added. It is well to test the reaction of the mixture, and if it is found to be acid, to render it neutral by adding a few drops of a solution of caustic soda or carbonate of soda. The whole is now boiled for half an hour, and filtered through absorbent cotton or filter paper. If the broth is to be kept, it should be placed in flasks and sterilized. The Loeffler blood serum mixture when ready is poured into tubes, which should be about four inches in length and two-thirds of an inch in diameter. These tubes should first be plugged with cotton and sterilized by dry heat at 150° C. for one hour. Care should be taken in filling the tubes to avoid the formation of air bubbles, as they leave a permanently uneven surface when the serum has been coagulated by heat. To prevent this, the end of the pipette or funnel which contains the serum should be inserted well into the test tube. About 2 c.c. are sufficient for each tube. The tubes, having been filled, are now to be coagulated and sterilized. The tubes are placed at the proper angle, and then kept for two hours at a temperature just below the boiling point. For this purpose a Koch serum coagulator or a double boiler serves best, though a steam sterilizer will suffice. If the latter is used, a wire frame must be arranged to hold the tubes at the proper inclination, and the degree of heat must be carefully watched, as otherwise the temperature may go too high, the serum actually boiled, and the culture medium thus spoiled. After sterilization by this process, the tubes containing the sterile, solidified blood serum can be placed in covered tin boxes and kept for months. The serum thus prepared is quite opaque and firm. A mixture of blood cells renders the serum darker, but it is not less useful.

The Swab for Inoculating Culture Tubes.

The swab to inoculate the serum is made as follows : A stiff, thin steel iron rod 6 inches in length is roughened at one end by a few blows of a hammer, and about this end a little absorbent cotton is firmly wound. Each swab is then placed in a separate glass tube, and the mouths of the tubes are plugged with cotton. The tubes and rods are then sterilized by dry heat at about 150° C. for one hour, and stored for future use. These cotton swabs have proved much more serviceable for making inoculations than platinum wire needles, especially in young children and in laryngeal cases. It is easier to use the cotton swab in such cases, and it gathers up so much more material for the inoculation that it has seemed more reliable.

For convenience and safety in transportation a "culture outfit" has been devised, which consists of a small wooden box containing a tube of blood serum, a tube holding a swab and a record blank. These "culture outfits" may be carried or sent by messenger or express to any place desired, and are kept at stations scattered throughout the city for the free use of physicians.

Directions for Inoculating Culture Tubes with the Exudate in Cases of Suspected Diphtheria.

The patient should be placed in a good light and, if a child, properly held. The swab is removed from its tube, and while the tongue is depressed with a spoon it is passed into the pharynx (if possible, without touching the tongue) and is rubbed gently but firmly against any visible membrane on the tonsils or in the pharynx, and then, without laying the swab down, it is immediately inserted in the blood serum tube, and the portion which has been previously in contact with the exudate is rubbed a number of times back and forth over the whole surface of the serum. This should be thoroughly done, but it is to be gently done, so as not to break the surface of the serum. The swab is replaced in its tube, and both tubes, their cotton plugs having been inserted, are returned to the box and sent to the collecting station. The blank forms of report which accompany each outfit should be completely filled out and forwarded to the station with the tubes.

Where there is no visible membrane (it may be present in the nose or pharynx) the swab should be thoroughly rubbed over the mucous membrane of the pharynx and tonsils, and in nasal cases, when possible, a culture should also be made from the nose. In little children, care should be taken not to use the swab when the throat contains food or vomited matter, as then the bacterial examination is rendered more difficult. Under no conditions should any attempt be made to collect the material shortly after the application of disinfectants (especially solutions of corrosive sublimate) to the throat. If any of these instructions have not been carried out, the fact should be carefully noted on the record blank.

The Examination of Cultures.

The culture tubes which have been inoculated, as described above, are kept in an incubator at 37° C. for twelve hours, and are then ready for examination. On inspection, it will be seen the surface of the blood serum is dotted with very numerous colonies, which are just visible. At this time no diagnosis can be made from simple inspection (if, however, the serum is found liquefied, or shows other evidences of contamination, the examination will probably be unsatisfactory). A microscopical preparation is now made by placing a tiny drop of water upon a clean cover glass, and then a platinum needle is nserted in the tube, and quite a large number of colonies are swept with it from the surface of the culture medium. The bacteria adherent to the needle are washed off in the drop of water previously placed on the cover glass, and smeared over its surface. The bacteria on the glass are then allowed to dry in the air. The cover glass is then passed quickly through the flame of a Bunsen burner or alcohol lamp 3 times in the usual way, covered with a few drops of Loeffler's solution of alkaline methyl blue, and left without heating for ten minutes. It is then rinsed off in clean water, dried and mounted in balsam.

In the great majority of cases, one of two pictures will be seen with the $\frac{1}{12}$ oil immersion lens ; either an enormous number of characteristic Loeffler bacilli with a moderate number of cocci, or a pure culture of cocci, mostly in pairs or short chains (see photographs). In a few cases there will be an approximately even mixture of Loeffler bacilli and cocci, and in others a great excess of cocci. Besides these, there will be occasionally met preparations, in which, with the cocci, there are mingled bacilli more or less resembling the Loeffler bacilli. These bacilli, which are pseudo-diphtheria bacilli (see photograph), are especially frequent in cultures from the nose.

In not more than 1 case in 20 will there be any serious difficulty in making the diagnosis, if the serum tube has been properly inoculated. In such a case, another culture must be made.

The Direct Microscopical Examination of the Exudate.

An immediate diagnosis, without the use of cultures, is often possible from a microscopical examination of the exudate. This is made by smearing a cover glass with a little exudate from the swab, drying, staining and examining it microscopically. This examination, however, is much more difficult, and the results more uncertain, than when the covers are prepared from cultures. The bacilli from the membrane are usually less typical in appearance than those found in cultures, and they are mixed with fibrin, pus and epithelial cells. They may also be very few in number in the parts reached by the swab, or bacilli may be met which closely resemble the Loeffler bacilli in appearance, but which differ greatly in growth and in other characteristics. When in a smear containing mostly cocci a few of these doubtful bacilli are present, it is impossible either to certainly exclude or make the diagnosis of diphtheria. Although in certain cases this immediate examination may be of the greatest value, it is not a method suitable for general use.

Characteristics of the Loeffler Bacillus.

When cover glass preparations made from the blood serum tubes are examined, the diphtheria bacillus are found to possess the following characteristics :

The diameter of the bacilli varies from 0.3 to 0.8 mm., and the length from 1.5 to 6.5 mm. They occur singly and in pairs (Photographs) and very infrequently in chains of 3 or 4. The rods are straight or slightly curved and usually are not uniformly cylindrical throughout their entire length, but are swollen at the ends, or pointed at the ends and swollen in the middle portion. Even from the same culture, different bacilli differ greatly in their size and shape. The 2 bacilli of a pair may lie with their long diameter in the same axis, or at an obtuse or an acute angle. The bacilli possess no spores, but have in them highly refractile bodies. They stain readily with the ordinary aniline dyes and retain their color after staining by Gram's method. With an alkaline solution of methyl blue, the bacilli, from blood serum especially, and from other media less constantly, stain in an irregular and extremely characteristic way (see photographs). The bacilli do not stain uniformly. Certain oval bodies situated in the ends, or in the central portions, stain much more intensely than the rest of the bacillus. Sometimes these highly stained bodies are thicker than the rest of the bacillus, again, they are thinner and surrounded by a more slightly stained portion. The bacilli seem to stain in this peculiar way at a certain period in their growth, so that only a portion of the organisms taken from a culture at any one time will show the characteristic staining. In old cultures, it is often difficult to stain the bacilli, and the staining, when it does occur, is frequently not at all characteristic.

Growth on Blood Serum.

If we examine the growth of the diphtheria bacillus in pure culture on blood serum, we will find at the end of ten to twelve hours little colonies of bacilli, which appear as pearl-gray or whitish-gray slightly raised points. The colonies when separated from each other may increase in forty-eight hours so that the diameter may be ¼ inch. The borders are usually somewhat uneven. Those colonies lying together fuse into one mass, especially if the serum is rather moist. During the first twelve hours, the colonies of the diphtheria bacilli about equal in size those of the streptococci; but after this time the diphtheria colonies become larger than those of the streptococci, nearly equalling those of the staphylococci. The diphtheria bacilli in their growth never liquefy the blood serum.

Growth on 1 Per Cent. Alkaline Glycerine Agar, and Method of Obtaining Pure Cultures.

It is frequently desired to obtain the diphtheria bacillus in pure culture. This is most readily accomplished by removing with a platinum needle a portion of the mixed growth of bacteria in a serum tube and lightly streaking it over the surface of the nutrient agar contained in a Petri dish.

Though the growth of the diphtheria bacilli upon agar is less certain and luxuriant than upon serum, the appearance of the colonies when examined under the microscope is more characteristic.

If the diphtheria colonies develop deep in the substance of the agar, they are usually round or oval, and, as a rule, present no extensions, but if near the surface, commonly from one but sometimes from both sides they spread out an apron-like extension which exceeds in surface area the rest of the colony. When the colonies develop entirely on the surface, they are more or less coarsely granular are nearly translucent, and usually have a darker centre. The edges are sometimes jagged and frequently shade off into a delicate lace-like fringe; at other times, the margins are more even and the colonies are nearly circular. With a high power lens, the edges show sprouting bacilli (see photographs). The colonies are gray or grayish-white by reflected light and pure gray with olive tint by transmitted light.

The growth of the diphtheria bacillus upon agar presents certain peculiarities which are of the utmost practical importance. While the bacilli from the majority of cases grow rather feebly, some grow luxuriantly. If a large number of the bacilli from a recent culture are implanted upon a properly prepared agar plate, a certain and fairly vigorous growth will always take place. If, however, the agar is inoculated with the exudate of a throat which contains but few Loeffler bacilli, no growth whatever of the bacilli may occur ; while the tubes of coagulated blood serum inoculated with the same exudate contain them abundantly. Again, agar prepared from broth made from different specimens of beef, or to which different peptones have been added, varies somewhat as to its suitability for the growth of the bacilli. Because of the uncertainty of obtaining a growth by the inoculation of agar with a few bacilli, or with bacilli of diminished vigor, agar is a far less reliable medium than blood serum for use in cultures made for diagnostic purposes, and is, therefore, not to be recommended. All agar should be tested by means of a pure culture of the diphtheria bacillus, before being used experimentally.

NOTE.—The agar is prepared by adding 1 per cent. of agar to the required quantity of broth. This broth is prepared in the same way as that used in the blood serum mixture already described, except that it contains no glucose. The agar must be thoroughly dissolved in the broth, and to accomplish this it is necessary to boil the mixture for from three to six hours. Before filtering, sufficient alkali must be added to make the agar slightly but distinctly alkaline. Finally, 6 per cent. of glycerine is added, and the mixture sterilized in flasks. When needed, it is melted and poured into sterilized Petri dishes in a thin layer.

Growth in Broth.

All the varieties of the Loeffler bacillus experimented with have grown in slightly alkaline broth with or without the addition of 1 per cent. glucose. The characteristic growth is one showing fine grains. These deposit along the sides and bottom of the tube, leaving the broth nearly clear. In some cultures, for twenty-four or forty-eight hours there is a more or less diffuse cloudiness and, exceptionally, a film forms over the surface of the broth. On shaking the tube, this film breaks up and slowly sinks to the bottom. All the varieties tested caused the alkaline broth to become acid, or, at least, distinctly less alkaline, within forty-eight hours.

ANIMAL INOCULATIONS AS A TEST OF VIRULENCE.

Animal experiments form the only reliable method of determining with certainty the virulence of the diphtheria bacillus. For this purpose, alkaline glucose broth cultures of forty-eight hours' growth should be used for the subcutaneous inoculation of guinea pigs. The amount injected may vary from ¼ to ½ per cent. of the body weight of the animal inoculated. In the great majority of cases when the bacilli are virulent, this amount causes death within seventy-two hours. In the autopsy the charateristic lesions described by Loeffler are found, namely : At the seat of inoculation there is a grayish focus surrounded by an area of congestion ; the subcutaneous tissues for an extensive area around are congested, and at times very œdematous ; the adjacent lymph nodes are swollen, and the serous cavities—especially the pleura—frequently contain an excess of fluid, usually clear, but at times turbid ; the lungs are usually congested. If the organs are subjected to microscopical examinations, the lesions described by Welch and Flexner (5), Babes (6) and others are found. There are numerous smaller and larger masses of necrotic cells, which are permeated by leucocytes. The heart and the voluntary muscular fibres usually show degenerative changes. The number of leucocytes in the blood is increased. From the area surrounding the point of injection, virulent bacilli may be obtained, but in distant areas and organs they are only occasionally found.

Bacilli which in cultures and in animal experiments have shown themselves to be character-istic may be regarded as certainly true diphtheria bacilli, and as capable of producing diphtheria in man under favorable conditions.

Original Investigations.

A large portion of the daily work in the laboratory has consisted in the routine examination of the cultures received each day. Besides this, however, a number of important questions have been studied experimentally, of which the most important are the following :

1. How much reliance can be placed on the bacteriological diagnosis made from the examina-tion of a culture inoculated with the exudations in the throat of a case of suspected diphtheria ?

2. If in cultures bacilli are found which possess the shape, size and staining characteristics of the diphtheria bacillus, can they, without further cultural or animal experiments, be considered as virulent diphtheria bacilli ?

3. What is the period of time during which virulent diphtheria bacilli remain in the throat after the disappearance of the exudate or pseudo-membrane ?

4. (a) What relation has the pseudo and the non-virulent diphtheria bacillus to the true virulent bacillus ? (b) Are virulent diphtheria bacilli ever present in the throats of healthy persons who have been in contact with diphtheria ?

5. To what degree is pseudo-diphtheria communicable ?

6. What are the means by which diphtheria is transmitted ?

7. How much reliance can be placed on the bacteriological diagnosis made from the examina-tion of a culture inoculated with the exudations in the throat of a case of suspected diphtheria ?

During the first few months, in order to test the results of the examinations and to make the liability to error as slight as possible, the following plan was adopted :

All cases in which the cultures yielded no diphtheria bacilli were turned over to special inspectors, who made, whenever possible, a second culture, and followed up the case during the illness, and for some time even after its recovery.

By means of the information thus obtained, the bacteriologists of the Department were able more and more surely to decide how far they could base an absolute diagnosis on a culture, especially when made by others. Many physicians, as well as the inspectors, gradually became so skilled in making inoculations that it was possible to rely certainly on the results obtained from the examination of their cultures, while, on the other hand, it was found that caution was necessary in accepting the inoculations of others, and in such cases a second culture was requested.

After a year's trial, the following conclusions have been arrived at :

The examination by a competent bacteriologist of the bacterial growth in a blood serum tube which has been properly inoculated and kept for fourteen hours at the body temperature, can be thoroughly relied on in cases where there is visible membrane in the throat, if the culture is made during the period in which the membrane is forming, and no antiseptic, especially no mercurial solution, has lately been applied.

In cases in which the disease is confined to the larynx or bronchi, and where, therefore, there is no visible exudate against which the swab can be rubbed, surprisingly accurate results can be obtained from the examination of cultures, but in a certain proportion of cases no diphtheria bacilli will be found in the first culture, and yet will be abundantly present in later ones, the bacilli having probably been coughed up more freely as the disease progressed. We believe, therefore, that absolute reliance for a diagnosis cannot be placed on a negative result in a single culture from the pharynx in purely laryngeal cases.

In nasal diphtheria a negative result may be obtained from a culture made from the throat, and yet the bacilli be found in cultures from the nose.

In making a diagnosis from a culture, it is essential to know the duration of the disease in the case from which it was made, because, although bacilli may remain present and alive in some throats for many weeks, it is, nevertheless, important to remember they may vanish early and suddenly, and that, therefore, the cultures cannot be certainly relied on after the membrane begins to disappear.

The use of antiseptics shortly before making the inoculation of a culture tube may render the culture useless for diagnosis. It has been found in a few instances that a culture made from a case of diphtheria, shortly after a thorough irrigation with a 1-4,000 solution of bi-chloride of mercury, gave no diphtheria bacilli, though one made just before and one made sometime later gave them abundantly. It is a curious fact that under such circumstances a vigorous growth of other organisms may take place.

The above conclusions are true only when the inoculations have been properly made, and, in judging cultures received from physicians in general, the greatest care must be taken. Some cultures are made carelessly, and some evidently without taking the pains to even read the instructions or to glance at the condition of the coagulated serum in the tube. If, therefore, when no diphtheria bacilli are found, the bacterial growth is scanty, the media dry or contaminated, or the inoculation in any way faulty, the case must be referred back for another culture. The second culture in these cases not infrequently contains the bacilli when the first did not.

The absence of bacilli in a culture proves the case to be one of false diphtheria only when it has been possible to make it under the proper conditions.

2. If, in cultures, bacilli are found, which possess the shape, size and staining characteristics of the diphtheria bacillus, can they, without further cultural or animal experiments, be considered as virulent diphtheria bacilli?

Since it is the custom in the Laboratory of the Health Department to make a bacteriological diagnosis in suspected cases of diphtheria, from the examination of the growth on the original blood serum tube without waiting for further cultural or animal experiments, it is of the greatest practical importance to ascertain to what extent bacilli appearing upon the serum in every way characteristic of the diphtheria bacilli, can be assumed to be virulent.

To test the virulence of bacilli, it is necessary to obtain them in pure culture, for otherwise it would be impossible to determine whether the changes produced in the inoculated animal were due to the supposed diphtheria bacilli or to other micro-organisms injected with them. It is further necessary to grow the bacilli in proper media, and to inoculate susceptible animals at a period when the growth of the bacilli in the media has reached its maximum. It is only when these precautions have been followed that accurate results will be obtained. The present almost uniform practice is to inoculate half-grown guinea pigs with from ¼ to ½ per cent. of their body weight of a forty-eight hours' culture of the bacilli grown at 37° C. in simple nutrient or glucose alkaline broth. It is important to remember that it is not safe to decide, because the growth derived from 1 bacillus is not virulent, that all the bacilli from that throat are not virulent. The cultures from several bacilli must be tried. The majority of those who have inoculated bacilli derived from pseudo-membranes and possessing the characteristics of the Loeffler bacilli, have found, as Loeffler did, that they were always virulent. The researches of Hofmann (15), Beck (16), and others, however, showing that in a certain number of healthy throats there were bacilli, which closely resembled the Loeffler bacillus, and yet were not virulent, stimulated others to subject the bacilli from large numbers of cases of suspected diphtheria to the test of animal inoculation.

In 1890, Roux and Yersin (17) published the results of some examinations as to the virulence of the bacilli obtained from 100 cases of diphtheria. 55 of these were fatal cases, and in all of them virulent bacilli were found, although in a few, together with many virulent bacilli, there were a few non-virulent ones. Among the 45 cases which recovered many were very mild, and in 10 of them they found no bacilli of sufficient virulence to cause the death of guinea pigs, when injected in moderate amount. From all of them, however, they obtained bacilli capable of causing inflammation in the guinea pig at the point of injection. This varied from slight, transient œdema to extensive necrosis. From further experiments they proved similar bacilli were capable under proper conditions to regain their virulence. They further showed in these milder cases, among many non-virulent or slightly virulent bacilli, there were usually a few virulent ones ; therefore, they believed, in most of these 10 cases fully virulent bacilli may have been present in the throat with the slightly virulent ones which by chance were used for the inoculations. In similar investigations carried on in a different locality, somewhat different results were obtained. Escherich (18) was unable to obtain from a large number of diphtheria cases studied any bacilli having the characteristics of the Loeffler bacillus which were not virulent, and only a few which, in injections of ¼ per cent. of the body weight of a forty-eight-hour bouillon culture, did not kill guinea pigs within forty-eight hours. Koplik (19), in New York, in testing the virulence of bacilli from mild cases of tonsillar diphtheria found them in every case fully virulent.

In Baltimore, Welch (20) and Abbott in 8 cases of diphtheria found the bacilli in every case fully virulent. In a later investigation, in which a large number of healthy and slightly inflamed throats were examined, Abbott (21) found in the cultures from 3, bacilli resembling the Klebs-Loeffler bacilli, but lacking virulence. These will be considered bacteriologically in connection with the pseudo-diphtheria bacilli, but the cases are of sufficient interest to be briefly quoted in the present consideration of the virulence of bacilli obtained from throats in which inflammatory lesions have appeared, which more or less resemble diphtheria.

Case 1—Adult, age 59. While in hospital, developed a laryngitis and pharyngitis. The uvula, tonsils and faucial pillars became swollen and œdematous, of an intense crimson red color, and covered with a thin, grayish white, slightly adherent exudate. In five days the patient completely recovered. Bacteriological examination showed abundant, apparently characteristic diphtheria bacilli, which, when inoculated, proved not to be virulent.

Case 2—Adult. Similar lesions to last ; well on ninth day. Bacteriological examination— abundant bacilli, in appearance similar to Klobs-Loeffler bacillus, but not virulent.

Case 3—Girl, age 11 years. Acute tonsilitis, with small white plug in one crypt. Quick recovery. Bacteriological examination, apparently characteristic Loeffler bacilli, but not virulent.

It must remain a matter of doubt whether some colonies from these cases would have been found to possess virulence if more had been tested as to this characteristic. These cases, as well as those of Roux and Yersin, show that now and then the bacilli from cases suspected to be diphtheria have little or no virulence.

Original Investigations.

In order to determine the virulence of the bacilli obtained in the ordinary routine examinations from suspected cases of diphtheria, blood serum cultures from 20 cases were selected, in which bacilli were found having the characteristic appearance of the virulent diphtheria bacilli. The cultures tested were selected before any information was possessed of the severity of the cases from which they were obtained, and were used for experiments on animals.

Virulence of the Bacilli Found in Twenty Cases of Throat Inflammation of Such a Character as to Arouse a Suspicion of Diphtheria.

SEVERITY.	WEIGHT OF GUINEA PIG GMS.	AMOUNT OF CULTURE INJECTED C. C.	DURATION OF LIFE AFTER INOCULATION.	PERSISTENCE OF LOEFFLER BACILLUS AFTER RECOVERY OF PATIENT.
1. Very mild case ; sick only four or five days..........	485	2	40 hours.....	14-19 days.
2. Moderately severe case ; subsequently contracted scarlet fever....................................	305	1	12 days......	
3. Mild case..	350	1	45 hours.....	24-32 days.
4. Mild case..	900	3	40 hours.....	
5. Mild case......,................................	405	1	40 hours.....	6 days.
6. Very mild case ; culture taken after disappearance of membrane	430	1.5	40 hours.....	13 days.
7. Very mild case...................................	410	1.5	40 hours.....	
8. Fatal case, and cause of severe case in mother........	435	1.33	40 hours.....	P. 16 days.
9. Mild case..	390	1.33	40 hours.....	P. 38-41 days.
10. Mild case ; adult ; never in bed....................	210	0.5	50 hours.....	P. 44 days.
11. Removed to Diphtheria Hospital ; severe case........	220	0.5	40 hours.....	
12. Rather mild case.................................	620	3.33	25 hours.....	P. 42 days.
13. Very mild case...................................	479	2	40 hours.....	P. 20-24 days.
14. Fatal case ; croup...............................	675	1.5	40 hours.....	
15. Fairly severe case, followed by measles..............	443	1.33	40 hours.....	P. 15-23 days.
16. Moderately severe case...........................	435	1.33	4 days.......	P. 15-19 days. R.
17. Moderately severe case...........................	510	1.66	40 hours.....	
18. Fatal case ; croup...............................	475	1.5	40 hours.....	
19. Very mild case...................................	500	1.66	40 hours.....	
20. Contracted from a mild case ; no membrane present...	250	1	40 hours.....	

We find, therefore, that the bacilli obtained from 20 cases of suspected diphtheria, ⅔ of which were very mild cases, proved in every case to be virulent, and in all but 3 fully so. If these results are considered in connection with those obtained by other American and

European observers, we must conclude, that for diagnostic purposes, all bacilli found in throat inflammations suspected to be diphtheria, which possess the morphological and cultural characteristics of the Loeffler bacilli, must be regarded as virulent, unless animal inoculations prove otherwise. Further, it should be remembered (as shown by Roux and Yersin, and as confirmed by others and by ourselves), that the absence of virulence in a culture derived from 1 bacillus is not sufficient to prove that cultures from other bacilli from the same case would not be virulent.

In 3 of the above cases, the cultures from the first colony selected were not virulent, while from others they were fully so.

3. What is the period of time during which virulent diphtheria bacilli remain in the throat after the disappearance of the exudate of pseudo-membrane?

If a piece of membrane be removed from the throat during the period of invasion of diphtheria and examined microscopically or by cultures the presence of abundant diphtheria bacilli will be noted. If, a few days later, when the membrane has begun to loosen, another bit be examined, the diphtheria bacilli will be found to be partly or at times wholly replaced by other microorganisms, mostly cocci. If, several days later, after the complete disappearance of the membrane, cultures be made from the mucous of the throat, it will be found the bacilli of diphtheria in many of the cases will have disappeared from the throat. This rule is not, however, without many exceptions, for it will be frequently found, days after the complete disappearance of the membrane and after the return of the throat to a healthy condition, fully virulent bacilli linger in the throat.

If we examine the researches of others regarding the matter, we find the following record in observations :

SEVERITY OF THE DIPHTHERIA IN THE CASE.	LENGTH OF TIME DURING WHICH THE BACILLI HAD PERSISTED AFTER THE DISAPPEARANCE OF THE EXUDATE WHEN THEY WERE TESTED AS TO THEIR VIRULENCE.	RESULTS OBTAINED FROM THE INOCULATION OF GUINEA PIGS.
Roux and Yersin (17).		
1. Mild case............	3 days...............	Guinea pig died, 24 hours.
2. Mild case	3 days...............	Fully virulent. Killed in a few hours.
3. Severe laryngeal case.	11 days...............	Guinea pig died in three days.
4. Severe case..........	14 days...............	Guinea pig. Fully virulent.
5. Mild case...........	9 days..............	Some colonies virulent ; some not virulent. For one week more, non-virulent bacilli were found.
6. Mild case............	7 days.......	Virulent and non-virulent colonies. For four days more, only non-virulent bacilli found.
7. Laryngeal case	15 days..............	On twelfth day, all virulent. On fifteenth, some virulent and some not virulent.
8. Severe case..........	2 months	Produced a slight local œdema only, when injected into guinea pigs.
Koplik (19).		
9. Mild case	14 days..............	Fully virulent.
10. Mild case...........	7 days..............	Virulent. A week later, the bacilli obtained were not virulent.
Loeffler (22).		
11. Moderate case........	8 days................	Fully virulent (this was twenty-fourth day of disease).

Escherich (18)—In a number of cases the Loeffler bacilli were found to persist after the disappearance of the membrane. In all of these, the bacilli were as virulent as those obtained at the height of the disease.

Morse (13)—In 25 cases found the average length of time the Loeffler bacillus remained in the throat after the disappearance of the membrane was ten days.

The average duration was the same for both nose and throat, although in some cases the bacilli were found in the throat much longer than in the nose, and vice versa. The bacilli disappeared in 1 case the day after the throat was clear, in another three days after, and in another four days after. The longest periods during which they persisted were twenty-two and thirty-seven days. The bacilli were tested from only 1 case, and these were fully virulent ten days after the disappearance of the membrane from the throat.

Tobiesen (23)—Found virulent diphtheria bacilli in the throats of 24 out of 46 patients at the time of their discharge from the hospital. The majority were children between 6 and 12 years. The following table gives the length of time after convalescence that the diphtheria bacilli were found :

SEVERITY OF CASE.	NUMBER OF CASES.	PERSISTENCE OF BACILLI AFTER DISAPPEARANCE OF MEMBRANE, AT TIME OF EXAMINATION AT DISCHARGE.	SEVERITY OF CASE.	NUMBER OF CASES.	PERSISTENCE OF BACILLI AFTER DISAPPEARANCE OF MEMBRANE, AT TIME OF EXAMINATION AT DISCHARGE.
Mild	1	4 days.	Moderate	1	10 days.
Moderate	5	4 "	Mild	1	10 "
"	4	5 "	Moderate	1	11 "
"	4	6 "	Severe	1	16 "
Mild	1	8 "	Moderate	1	22 "
Moderate	1	8 "	"	1	31 "
"	1	9 "			
Severe	1	9 "		24	153 days.

Average..6.924

In the 22 of Tobiesen's cases in which the bacilli were not found, the length of stay in hospital of the patients after convalescence was about the same. Tobiesen's studies indicate that the existence of throat lesions render the conditions more favorable for the persistence of bacilli. The virulence of the bacilli was proven in 19 out of 24. In 16 cases the guinea pigs died within a period of fifty hours, and the autopsies showed typical lesions ; in 2, local necrosis developed, followed by death in 1 animal and recovery in the other. In the last case the animal developed paralysis five weeks after the local symptoms had disappeared. From these results he draws the following conclusions :

In 19 out of the 24 persistent cases, the Loeffler bacilli proved virulent, and the probability is they were also virulent in the 5 not tested. In other words, ½ of the patients who are allowed to leave the hospital under the usual conditions carry virulent bacilli in their throats, and are capable of giving diphtheria to others. Clinical investigation alone can decide the frequency with which these convalescent cases infect others. This investigation must be carried on with great caution. In the 24 investigated by Tobiesen, he excluded those where numerous cases had occurred in the house besides the ones under investigation. Among those remaining he discovered 1 where the convalescent child was the almost certain cause of diphtheria in another.

Original Investigations.

In order to test the virulence of the bacilli in the throats of convalescent cases, they were obtained in pure culture from the healthy throats of 15 convalescent diphtheria cases and used for the inoculation of the guinea pigs. The following table gives the results of these experiments:

Case No.	Severity of the Diphtheria in the Case.	The Bacilli Tested Persisted after Recovery for—	Virulence.			Persistence from Inception of Disease.	
			Weight guinea pig, gms.	Amount Injected, c. c.	Life of guinea pig after Injection.	Still present, days.	Absent, days.
1	Rather severe case.........	8 days........	392	1.33	60–70 hours...........	13	17
2	Mild case.................	10 "	250	0.5	8 days..............	12	19
3	"	12 "	290	1.25	11 "	?	?
4	Severe case...............	18 "	229	1.00	9 "	21	30
5	Moderate case............	6 "	549	1.25	14 "	10	22
6	Mild case	33 "	*226	1.00	Extensive necrosis with final recovery	38	..
7	Very mild case	12 "	440	1.5	40 hours.............	14	22
8	Mild case	8 "	310	2.00	40 "	16	20
10	Very mild case	25 "	505	1.66	40 "	30	?
11	Very mild case (nasal)	10 "	253	2.00	40 "	10	?
12	Mild case.................	6 "	490	1.66	40 "	24	?
13	"	8 "	450	1.33	40 "	13	20
14	"	12 "	367	1.33	40 "	19	..
15	Fairly severe case	26 "	347	1.33	5 days..............	35	44
16	Mild case.................	50 "	410	3.00	2 "	56	..

In each case, in testing the virulence of the bacilli derived from it, we employed the last culture or the next to the last culture made from it in which the bacilli were found to be present. The results in these 15 cases tested, as well as in those before recorded by others, prove conclusively that the bacilli, which in a certain proportion of cases persist in the throat after an attack of diphtheria, are always virulent for some time. In the exceptional cases in which the bacilli persist for a very long time, it is found they occasionally loose their virulence a few days before their final disappearance, while in other cases they retain their virulence to the end. That the cases themselves are not so liable to spread diphtheria is probably because of the relatively small number of bacilli present in convalescent throats as compared with the number found in those showing the lesions of diphtheria.

During the last six months completed observations have been made in 605 cases of diphtheria as to the length of time during which the Loeffler bacilli persist. In these cases cultures were made at the beginning of the disease, and then again at short intervals after the complete disappearance of the exudate, until the throat was found to be free of diphtheria bacilli. The custom was to make the second culture three days after the complete disappearance of the membrane, and then, when necessary, to make further cultures about every fourth or fifth day. In 304 of these 605 cases the diphtheria bacilli disappeared within three days after the complete disappearance of the exudate ; in 301 cases the diphtheria bacilli persisted for a longer time, viz. : in 176 cases, for seven days ; in 64 cases, for twelve days ; in 36 cases, for fifteen days ; in 12 cases, for three weeks ; in 4 cases, for four weeks ; in 4 cases, for five weeks, and in 2 cases for nine weeks after the time when the exudate had to all appearances completely disappeared from the upper air passages.

4. (a) What relation has the pseudo and the non-virulent diphtheria bacillus to the true, virulent bacillus?

In 1888 Hofmann published the results of the bacteriological examinations of a number of diseased and healthy throats, which for a time threw doubt on the specific character of the Loeffler diphtheria bacillus. Further research has entirely dispelled the confusion which his discoveries seemed to make, but the results of these studies and of similar ones on the virulent and non-virulent bacilli are of such practical importance in relation to the bacteriological diagnosis of cases of suspected diphtheria that a detailed account of the work of the subsequent investigators as well as that of the Health Department will be presented.

Hofmann's (15) results were similar to those of Loeffler, in that he found the virulent bacillus in all of 8 cases of true diphtheria, but in further search he was suprised to find in the throats of 26 out of 45 persons, none of whom was suffering from diphtheria, a bacillus which very closely resembled the Loeffler bacillus. Some of these persons were suffering from scarlet fever, measles or some other disease, while many were entirely healthy. The bacilli from a number of these healthy throats were obtained in pure culture and inoculated into animals. The majority had no virulence whatever. The bacilli from the different cases varied somewhat in their characteristics. Some in appearance, manner of staining and growth on media, seemed identical with the Loeffler bacillus, while others presented slight but constant differences. Between the extremes were many gradations.

Those bacilli which did not possess all the characteristics of the virulent bacillus differed in the following respects. They were shorter, thicker, and more uniform in size. On agar, they grew in whiter and thicker colonies, whose circumference was more circular and less notched. They also grew at a lower temperature than the virulent bacilli (20° to 22° C.).

Hofmann was undecided whether all of these bacilli were really Loeffler diphtheria bacilli, which had lost their virulence, or whether they were a different species of bacteria and of a saprophytic nature. He was also undecided whether, even among these non-virulent bacilli there might not be included different species. Hofmann's death prevented further attempts on his part to solve this problem, and different investigators since that time have been divided in their opinions ; some taking the view that these bacilli were derived from true Loeffler bacilli, having merely lost their virulence ; others, that they were a different species, having no connection with the Loeffler bacillus ; and still others consider the matter as undecided. The results of two other important series of investigations should be considered here ; those of Roux and Yersin and those of Escherich.

Roux and Yersin found in a hospital for children in Paris, where cases of diphtheria occurred from time to time, that 15 out of 45 children contained in their healthy throats non-virulent bacilli resembling the Loeffler bacillus. In a French village, where no diphtheria had been present for a long time, they made cultures from the healthy throats of 59 children living in a school. In 26 of these non-virulent bacilli were found.

In an examination of the throats of 10 attendants in a diphtheria hospital non-virulent bacilli were found once. Thus, in 114 healthy throats the non-virulent bacilli were found 42 times. In all of these throats the bacilli were present in very small numbers. They found the same bacilli twice in 6 children with mild sore throats, and 5 times in 7 children sick with measles. It should be noted that these examinations were made chiefly in a hospital and in a school, both for children. In both of these the children were confined together for considerable periods of time, and the direct transmission of the bacilla from one throat to another would be likely to occur. The unusually large percentage of children in which they were found might thus be accounted for.

The bacilli found, when studied in pure culture, differed somewhat from each other. The majority were identical in all their characteristics with the Loeffler bacillus, except as to their lack of virulence. The minority resembled those described by Hofmann, being shorter and thicker and growing at a lower temperature than the characteristic Loeffler bacilli. They made the important observation that the non-virulent bacilli which they tested, when grown in broth, caused the same changes in the reaction as the virulent forms, namely, from alkaline to acid in forty-eight to seventy-two hours, and later, back again to alkaline in the course of some weeks. These changes were found to occur even more rapidly in the cultures of the non-virulent than of the virulent bacilli. Roux and Yersin regarded the occasional slight differences in growth, shape and staining as too slight and inconstant to distinguish the virulent from the non-virulent bacilli. Animal experiments alone sufficed to determine the question of virulence, and they regarded as arbitrary a division founded on the reaction of the guinea pig to inoculation ; since they found bacilla from cases of diphtheria may possess every degree of virulence, from those which cause death within twenty-four hours to those which caused only a temporary œdema. With such variations it is a difficult matter to determine what should be the proper line of division between the virulent and the non-virulent bacilli.

To fully prove these bacilli belong to the same species, they believe it is necessary to derive non-virulent bacilli from the virulent ones, and to give virulence to those entirely lacking it.

They found it was possible to produce an attenuation of the virulence of the bacilli in a number of ways. For instance, if a current of sterile air is kept passing through a broth culture of diphtheria bacilli, maintained at a temperature of 39½° C, after about two weeks some of the bacilli begin to lose their virulence, and at the end of about four weeks all of the bacilli have lost all of their virulence and produce non-virulent cultures. A little while after losing their virulence, bacilli remaining in the culture died.

They also found that if from time to time cultures were made from dried bits of membrane, a period finally came when the bacilli, although alive had become non-virulent. Thus they had fulfilled the first condition.

The attempt to restore to bacilli the virulence which they had entirely lost was not so successful. They found it possible to greatly increase the virulence of bacilli by injecting them together with a virulent culture of the streptococcus of erysipelas. The bacilli obtained from animals which had succumbed to this double inoculation were found to have fully regained their virulence. Roux and Yersin were unable, on the other hand, to give back virulence to those bacilli which had been completely robbed of their virulence by the above methods, or to those which had no virulence when obtained from the throat. Thus, of the two proofs necessary to establish the identity of the virulent and non-virulent forms, they had obtained the first fully, the second only partially.

As additional proof of the identity of the virulent and non-virulent bacilli, they brought forward the fact that they found the latter more frequently in patients recently convalescent from true diphtheria than in those who had never had the disease, and that the bacilli which had artificially been deprived of their virulence, frequently were changed in other respects, so as to resemble in all ways the bacilli which were originally lacking in virulence. From their studies, they concluded the non-virulent and virulent bacilli were one and the same species of bacteria.

If we now turn to the work of Escherich, we find results which tend to show the virulent and some of the non-virulent bacilli are different species of bacteria.

He first lays stress on the methods to be employed in testing the virulence. He advises the animal inoculations be made always from broth cultures, which have been grown for forty-eight hours at $37\frac{1}{2}°$ C, and that the amount of the culture be regulated by the size of the animal. With these precautions, he found the bacilli from every case of diphtheria examined to be fully virulent, and in a few cases, where he obtained characteristic bacilli from the healthy throats of persons exposed to diphtheria, he found them also to be virulent.

Escherich did indeed find in a moderate number of throats of persons not suffering from diphtheria a bacillus similar to those described by Hofmann. Thus, in Munich he found this non-virulent bacillus in 2 throats out of 70, and in Grez, in 11 out of 250, or 13 times in 320 cases. These bacilli, however, all possessed certain cultural and morphological characteristics which were sufficient to separate them from the virulent bacilli. They were, as in some described by Hofmann, plumper and shorter than the Loeffler bacilli and more uniform in size. The growth on agar was more luxuriant and whiter than is the case with the diphtheria bacilli. He noticed two new points of difference which seemed to him important. The non-virulent or pseudo-diphtheria bacilli, when spread on a cover glass, lie in parallel rows, while the virulent diphtheria bacilli lie at every angle and the most varied positions. The second difference was still more marked. He found, as had all others who had noticed this point, that the virulent bacilli in their growth in alkaline bouillon changed the reaction of the bouillon to acid in the course of forty-eight hours. The amount of acid formed differed in different cultures, and had no relation to the degree of virulence. He then noticed the pseudo-diphtheria bacilli always made the bouillon more alkaline instead of acid. Therefore, if at the end of forty-eight hours litmus was added to the different bouillon cultures, it turned red in the virulent ones and blue in the pseudo-diphtheritic non-virulent ones. Although this will be referred to again, it should be noticed this difference in reaction was not found by Roux and Yersin in the cultures of the non-virulent bacilli tested by them.

Escherich, in conclusion, states his position as follows :

" Since we have found constant cultural differences between the true and the pseudo-diphtheria bacilli, we can give the pseudo-diphtheria bacilli no diagnostic value. We do not find it to be a frequent inhabitant of the mouth. Chronic throat inflammations and measles seem to render the throat more liable to the invasion."

He did not find, as Roux and Yersin and Fraenkel had, that it was possible to determine from the abundance of the colonies of bacilli present whether they were composed of virulent or non-virulent bacilli.

If we review the remaining literature of this subject we find some investigators have been led by the results to adopt views similar to those of Roux and Yersin, others to those of Escherich, and still others have been forced to content themselves with the position of Hofmann, viz. : that we are not yet in a position to affirm whether all these bacilli are of one or of different species of bacteria.

Up to the present time, the results, so far as they are known to the writers, are given in the following table :

	VON HOFMANN (15).	LOEFFLER (3).
Morphology	Some bacilli identical with those of Loeffler, others were shorter, thicker and more uniform in size.	Somewhat larger than virulent bacilli and more tendency to produce swollen ends.
Growth in bouillon and reaction	Similar to virulent.	Similar to virulent.
Growth on blood serum.	Sometimes identical with Loeffler bacilli ; again, found in larger and somewhat whiter colonies.	Similar to virulent.
Growth on agar	Grows most luxuriantly and spreads more on the surface. May become of a dirty brown color in central part of colonies.	Colonies had less jagged edges and were of a whiter hue.
Frequency met with	In 45 throats, comprising some healthy and some the seat of non-diphtheritic inflammations they were found in 26.	Once with virulent bacilli from a case of diphtheria.
Opinion as to the nature of the bacilli	Is doubtful whether these non-virulent bacilli belong to the same species as the virulent diphtheria bacilli, or whether they are of a different species.	Believes them to be of a different species, but only to be separated by animal cultures.

	ESCHERICH (18).	BECK (16).
Morphology	Bacilli shorter, plumper and more uniform in size. When a drop of bouillon culture is smeared on a cover glass, the bacilli are found to lie in parallel rows.	Shorter, plumper bacilli as a rule, but some more like virulent bacilli.
Growth in bouillon and reaction	More luxuriant growths, with tendency to cause cloudiness ; when grown in neutral litmus bouillon, the litmus turns blue after two or three days.	Quicker and more luxuriant in growth.
Growth on blood serum	Fairly characteristic, but apt to be a more luxuriant and whiter growth.	Somewhat more luxuriant, and of a more yellow color.
Growth on agar	Grows more luxuriantly and spreads more on surface ; may become brownish in color after some days.	Colonies less jagged on margin and more yellow in hue.
Frequency met with	In Munich, in 2 out of 70 ; in Graz, in 11 out of 250 healthy throats and those the seat of non-diphtheritic lesions examined. 13 in 320	In 66 well children, found in 22 ; in 41 non-diphtheritic affections, in 14, or in a total of 107, found them in 36. Also, along with virulent bacilli in true diphtheria.
Opinion as to the nature of the bacilli	Believes that they have no relation to the virulent diphtheria bacilli, and that they can be separated pretty accurately by cultural differences.	Believed that the non-virulent forms found by him were of a different species from the virulent, and were saprophytic in nature.

	KOPLIK (19), FIRST PAPER.	KOPLIK (19), SECOND PAPER.
Morphology	Short, plump, uniform in size ; take a more uniform stain.	Identical in form and size with virulent and characteristic stain.
Growth in bouillon and reaction	More luxuriant, cloudy at first, afterward clearing, with abundant deposit ; bouillon acid after forty-eight hours.	Cloudy ; less abundant growth in bouillon to which glucose has been added ; bouillon alkaline after forty-eight hours.
Growth on blood serum	More luxuriant and spreading.	More luxuriant, opaque and whiter growth.
Growth on agar	More luxuriant and spreading.	More luxuriant, opaque and whiter growth.
Frequency met with	In 4 mild throat inflammations.	In 2, following true attack of diphtheria. For first three weeks found virulent bacilli ; then for two weeks there were non-virulent forms.
Opinion as to the nature of the bacilli	Are of a different species from Loeffler bacilli.	

	ROUX AND YERSIN (2).	ABBOTT (3).
Morphology...........	Majority identical with virulent bacilli. The minority of shorter, plumper and more uniform variety.	Bacilli from 3 cases were identical with virulent forms; from 1 they were larger than the virulent average.
Growth in bouillon and reaction...........	Characteristic, except for slight cloudiness. Changes of broth were same as in virulent forms, but somewhat more rapid.	Growth in bouillon same as in virulent forms, except the changes from alkaline to acid, and, later, back again to alkaline, were more rapid than in case of virulent bacilli.
Growth on blood serum...	Same as in virulent.	Characteristic.
Growth on agar........	Same as in virulent, varying within the limits noticed in different virulent cultures.	Two of 4 characteristic; 1 more luxuriant in growth, and 1 giving colonies with darker central portion.
Frequency met with....	In 104 healthy children's throats found 41 times; 10 adults, once; in 6 mild throat inflammations, twice; in 7 sick with measles, five times.	Four times in 53 throats. Some healthy, others the seat of moderately severe inflammations.
Opinion as to the nature of the bacilli........	Believed the non-virulent to be of the same species as the virulent; they were simply an attenuated form......	In doubt.
Note..................	....	The bacillus growing more luxuriantly on agar gave a dirty brown growth on potato.

	FRAENKEL (24).	MARTIN (10).
Morphology.............	Identical with virulent forms.............	Short, plump bacilli.
Growth in bouillon and reaction...........	Characteristic.....................	
Growth on blood serum...	Characteristic......................	
Growth on agar..........	Characteristic......................	More moist, luxuriant and whiter. Grow at room temperature.
Frequency met with....	In number of healthy conjunctive and in some cases of mild tonsilitis and with virulent bacilli in diphtheria. Figures not given......................	In quite a number of diphtheria cases running in mild course.
Opinion as to the nature of the bacilli........	Believes the virulent and non-virulent to be of same species, and includes under non-virulent some causing local reaction......................	An attenuated form of the virulent diphtheria bacillus.

If we inspect closely the descriptions of the non-virulent bacilli, we find there seems to be two forms which stand out distinctly as separate varieties with which the others can be grouped.

First—Bacilli which are in all respects, except that they lack virulence, identical with the Loeffler bacillus, and which, like it, produce an acid in their growth in broth cultures.

Second—Bacilli which are shorter, plumper and more uniform in size than the Loeffler bacilli, and which produce an alkali in their growth in broth cultures.

As we look over the tables, we see that some observers have chanced to find one of these varieties, some the other, and some both. This has led to the present confusion.

Original Investigations.

In order to study these various bacilli, and to clear up, if possible, some of the questions connected with their classification, cultures were made upon blood serum from 330 healthy throats.

When any of the varieties of bacilli described above were discovered in the cultures, they were isolated, and in the great majority of cases, tested as to their virulence on guinea pigs. The results of these studies are given in the tables below. The bacilli formed may be divided into three groups :

(1) Bacilli identical with the Loeffler diphtheria bacillus in growth, producing acid in bouillon, but having no virulence.

(2) Bacilli not having all the characteristics of the Loeffler bacillus in growth producing alkali in bouillon, and having no virulence.

(3) Virulent Loeffler diphtheria bacilli, characteristic in growth, producing acid in bouillon.

Table Showing Results of Cultures Made from the Throats of Healthy Persons where there had been no History Obtained of Direct Contact with Diphtheria.

FROM WHERE.	TOTAL CASES.	VIRULENT CHARACTERISTIC DIPHTHERIA BACILLI.	NON-VIRULENT CHARACTERISTIC DIPHTHERIA BACILLI.	NON-VIRULENT PSEUDO-DIPHTHERIA BACILLI.
New York Dispensary, by Dr. J. H. Huddleston......	Nos. 1 to 151	3	12	21
Northern Dispensary.........	152 to 163	..	..	..
Vanderbilt Clinic	164 to 189	..	2	2
Throughout the city..........................	190 to 193	..	4	..
College of Physicians and Surgeons—Students.	194 to 242	..	2	3
New York F. H. Dispensary.................	243 to 257	..	..	1
Orthopedic Hospital (through kindness of Dr. Chappell) :				
Female Ward..........................	258 to 267	} ..	} 3	} ..
Male Ward.............................	268 to 275			
New York Foundling Hospital, By Dr. Adams..............	276 to 330	5	1	..
Totals..................	330	8	24	27

A Comparative Table of—

CASE NO. AND SOURCE.	NON-VIRULENT DIPHTHERIA BACILLI.		PSEUDO-DIPHTHERIA BACILLI.	
	N. Y. 66, Throat. (1)	N. Y. 72, Throat. (2)	P. & S. 30, Throat. (1)	N. Y. 101, Throat. (2)
Examination of bacilli in primary culture	Abundant large characteristic diphtheria bacilli.	Abundant characteristic diphtheria bacilli.	Abundant short even stained bacilli (see photograph of pseudo-diphtheria bacilli).	Abundant short even stained bacilli (pseudo-diphtheria).
Growth in pure culture on serum at 37½ C......	Characteristic appearance of colonies.	Characteristic.	Fairly characteristic appearance of colonies.	Characteristic appearance of colonies.
Agar	Fairly typical colonies.	Not typical colonies.	Coarsely granular colonies, with jagged, rough borders, and of about equal thickness throughout, brownish hue by transmitted light.	Fairly typical; more heavily pigmented and uniformly thick than is characteristic of the virulent bacilli; colonies nearly circular, with even borders.
Growth in neutral glucose broth..	Characteristic. Acid at end of forty-two hours.	Not characteristic; broth cloudy for two days; acid at end of forty-eight hours.	Typical growth in rather coarse grains; alkaline reaction end of forty-eight hours.	Formation of thin pellicle and slight diffuse cloudiness; alkaline reaction at end forty-eight hours.
Virulence in guinea pigs	Guinea pig, 216 gms., 1.33 c.c.; no reaction.	Guinea pig, 164 gms., 1.33 c.c.; no reaction.	Guinea pig, 405 gms., 3 c.c.; no reaction.	Guinea pig, 400 gms., 2 c.c.; no reaction.
Clinical notes.....	Bronchitis; diphtheria in house; three weeks previous.	Intest. catarrh; no history of contagion.	Healthy throat.	Bronchitis; no history of contagion.
Sex................	Female, one year.	Female, fifteen mos.	Twenty-seven years.	Male, ten years.

In the above table we find 24 cases containing bacilli possessing all the characteristics of the Loeffler bacilli except that of virulence, namely :

Nos. 7, 33, 52, 63, 66, 72, 103, 105, 110, 114, 124, 132, 188, 189, 190, 191, 192, 193, 198, 212, 258, 259, 260, 297.

These bacilli were abundant in the primary cultures from 17 cases and present in small numbers only in the cultures from 7.

They were on the average a little longer than the virulent bacilli from the cases of suspected diphtheria examined on the same days. In broth, the bacilli from 13 of the 24 cases grew characteristically, while from 6 they caused a more or less dense cloudiness. It was found, however, that sometimes the virulent bacilli produced the same effect though never to the same degree as the bacilli from case 191. In 5 cases the bacilli were not grown in broth. In all the cases in which broth cultures were made (19) the bacilli produced acid in their growth. When their acid producing power was compared with that of an equal number of virulent cultures no marked difference could be noted. Some virulent bacilli were found to produce more acid than the non-virulent ones, while others produced less.

Upon blood serum, the bacilli grew in a manner characteristic of the Loeffler bacillus.

Upon agar, the bacilli from 11 cases grew as the virulent bacilli usually grow, while from 7 they grew in a less typical manner, but always in ways seen exceptionally in the virulent form. Guinea pigs were inoculated with the bacilli from 15 cases. The lack of virulence in the bacilli from the remaining 9 cases was taken for granted from the close association with the 15 tested.

For this purpose half-grown guinea pigs were employed, and they were inoculated under the skin with ½ per cent. of their weight of a forty-eight hour broth culture. In only 1 animal was there any appreciable reaction, and in this the local induration caused passed away within four days. A very slight degree of immunity was given to some of the pigs by the injection.

Two hundred and eighty of the 330 healthy persons from whose throats cultures were made were children under twelve, while 50 were adults. In 24 of these characteristic but non-virulent bacilli were found, and in only 9 of the 24 were there present noticeable pathological changes in the throat, such as enlarged tonsils. The bacilli persisted in 4 of the throats for four weeks, in 1 for three weeks, in 3 for two weeks, and in some of the others for shorter periods.

Column III. of the table shows that in 27 cases bacilli were found corresponding to those described by Hofmann and Escherich and photographed by Koplik (19). These were smaller, shorter, thicker and more uniform in size than the Loeffler bacilli, and always formed alkali in their growth in broth. These bacilli were never virulent in animals. Guinea pigs were inoculated with large amounts (½ to 1 per cent. of their weight) of broth cultures of bacilli, obtained from 8 cases, without showing any reaction.

As is shown in Column I. of the table, virulent diphtheria bacilli were found in 8 of the 330 cases. They were, in all probability, derived from mild cases of unrecognized diphtheria or from healthy children who were carrying the bacilli in their throats. The number of such infected children is indicated by the results of studies described in the following pages.

4 (b). Are virulent diphtheria bacilli ever present in the throats of healthy persons who have been brought in contact with diphtheria?

The search for the origin of obscure cases of diphtheria has revealed the fact that it is possible for the human throat to become the habitat of the virulent Loeffler bacillus without any visible lesions resulting. Thus, Loeffler (3) found the virulent bacillus once, Fraenkel (24) twice, and Escherich (18) found it in several cases. In one of Escherich's cases the history is so significant as to be worth repeating. It was noticed among the children coming under the care of a certain apparently healthy nurse a number of cases of diphtheria were developing. A bacteriological examination being made, her throat was found to contain very numerous virulent diphtheria bacilli. These remained present and virulent for weeks. A similar and interesting case is reported by Feer (25). In a diphtheria epidemic occurring in a hospital ward, due to a single infection, the throats of 7 children became infected. The infection caused fatal diphtheria in 4, an acute angina without membrane in 2, and no symptoms whatever in 1. In all of these the bacilli were abundant and equally virulent. Many similar examples have been met with by one of us (Park).

A very interesting investigation has been carried on to determine how frequently the throats of healthy children become infected in families where one is sick with diphtheria, and where little or no isolation is possible.

As will be seen by the following tables, the throats of the healthy children of 14 families, in which 1 or more of the other members had diphtheria, were examined. There were in all 48 healthy children. In 50 per cent. of these diphtheria bacilli were found, 40 per cent. developed later, to a greater or less extent, the lesions of diphtheria. In considering the high percentage of cases in which this virulent Loeffler bacillus was found, it must be remembered in these families the conditions were the best possible for the transmission of the contagion.

In numerous instances cultures have been made from the throats of healthy children in families where the diphtheria case was well isolated, in such cases the bacilli have been found in less than 10 per cent. of the children.

FAMILY.	NUMBER OF CASES EXAMINED ASIDE FROM THE ORIGINAL CASE OF DIPHTHERIA.	LOEFFLER BACILLI.		REMARKS.
		FOUND IN.	NOT FOUND IN.	
A.	1	..	1	Isolation partial.
B.	3	3	..	{ No isolation ; all three cases subsequently developed diphtheria.
C.	2	1	1	No isolation.
D.	1	1	..	"
E.	3	1	2	"
F.	4	1	3	Isolation partial.
G.	5	3	2	"
H.	4	3	1	No isolation.
I.	4	1	3	Isolation partial.
J.	8	3	5	"
K.	4	1	3	"
L.	3	1	1	"
M.	5	3	2	"
N.	1	1	..	No isolation.
14	48	24	24	

Of the above cultures in which the Loeffler bacilli were found, in 6 the virulence was tested in the usual way. The results are stated in the following table :

FAMILY NO.	CASE NO.	AMOUNT BOUILLON CULTURE INOCULATED.	WEIGHT GUINEA PIG GMS.	VIRULENCE.	CLINICAL HISTORY.
B.	1	1.33 c.c.	337	Died in 40 hours.	{ Developed fatal diphtheria one day after culture was taken.
G.	2	1 "	205	Died in 44 hours.	{ Developed tonsilar diphtheria two days after culture was taken.
H.	3	1.33 "	202	Died in 48 hours.	No subsequent development of diphtheria.
K.	4	1.33 "	300	Died in 40 hours.	" "
M.	5	1.66 "	490	Died in 40 hours.	" "
N.	6	1 "	250	Died in 40 hours.	" "

It may be interesting to detail here 2 instances out of many observed in which the virulent bacilli of diphtheria derived from healthy throats have been the cause of diphtheria in others.

1. A child was admitted into a hospital ward in an anæmic condition and with a chronic coryza. Five days later 4 children in his neighborhood developed diphtheria. 2 of these died. In seeking the cause of the diphtheria, suspicion was directed to the child by a slight nasal discharge. Bacteriological examination showed this secretion contained many diphtheria bacilli. On further examination, it was found the child came from a family in which three weeks before there had been a case of diphtheria.

2. In a family of 8 children 1 child sickened with diphtheria and a second child, a baby, was sent to a neighbor. The next day cultures showed this baby, as well as 2 of the other children, all of whom were apparently healthy, were infected with diphtheria bacilli. The 3 apparently healthy, but infected, children, as well as the sick one were at once quarantined, but already 1 of the family to which the baby had been sent had contracted diphtheria from it.

The practical value of bacteriological examinations of the throats of healthy children in families where isolation has not been carried out in the first days is further shown by the fact that those children in whom the bacilli are found are extremely apt to develop diphtheria in the course of a few days, when no cleansing treatment is adopted, while they seem much less liable to do so if kept under treatment.

The detection of the virulent bacilli in throats prevents the dissemination of diphtheria by allowing us to isolate those infected.

A very striking instance of this was the following: In a family of 4 children 1 was sick with diphtheria. The Department Inspector found 3 other children in the same bed with the sick one, who was constantly spitting upon and soiling the bedclothes. He made cultures from these 3 children, whose throats appeared healthy, as well as from the sick one ; all contained abundant characteristic Loeffler bacilli (these were later shown to be virulent by the inoculation of guinea pigs). When the Inspector visited the same family three days later he found 2 of the previously healthy children had meanwhile sickened and died, and that the third was severely ill. This child finally recovered.

From the observation detailed above, we cannot escape the conclusion that all members of an infected household should be regarded as under suspicion, and in those cases where isolation is not enforced, the healthy as well as the sick should be prevented from mingling with others until cultures from the throat have shown the absence of bacilli, or a sufficient lapse of time gives the presumption that they are not carriers of the contagion.

SUMMARY AND CONCLUSIONS ON DIPHTHERIA BACILLI IN HEALTHY THROATS.

We have found that children, and to a less extent adults, who are brought in direct contact with true cases of diphtheria very often receive the diphtheria bacilli into their throats, and that these bacilli may persist and develop in these throats for days or weeks. In some cases we have found that true diphtheria followed the appearance of the bacilli in the respiratory passages, while in others no disease developed, though they might be the source of diphtheria in others. The examination of the throats of 330 healthy persons in whom no contact with diphtheria was known, revealed the presence of virulent bacilli in but 8 persons, 2 of whom later developed diphtheria.

We must conclude then that virulent diphtheria bacilli are to be found in the throats of a small proportion of healthy persons throughout the city, and that they have been derived either directly from diphtheria cases or from those who have been in contact with them. The examinations of the throats of the 330 healthy persons showed that in 24 bacilli existed in every way identical with the Loeffler bacillus, except that they were not virulent in animals. As the bacilli in cases of true diphtheria are known to gradually lose their virulence, and as this loss of virulence can be caused artificially, it seems to the writers that these bacilli, characteristic except as to virulence, should be regarded as true diphtheria bacilli which have lost their virulence.

The examination of the same throats showed that in 27 there were bacilli present which were so uniform in their peculiarities as to staining, size, shape and the production of an alkali instead of an acid, that there seems to us to be even more reason to separate them from the diphtheria bacillus than there is, for example, to separate the colon bacillus from that of typhoid.

We have never found bacilli possessing these peculiarities to be virulent, nor have they seemed to have any connection with diphtheria. It seems to us that to these bacilli alone the name pseudo-diphtheria bacillus should be given.

The few bacilli which do not seem to come under either of these divisions must await further study before being classified.

5. *To what Degree is Pseudo-diphtheria Communicable?*

In the general circular issued by the Department, it was announced that cases which bacteriologically proved to be false diphtheria would not be kept under the supervision of the Department. Some who approve heartily of the rest of the work of the Board in its dealings with diphtheria believe in this step it has made a mistake, and that the pseudo-diphtheria cases, though less contagious than the true, are yet sufficiently so as to render isolation necessary. From the experience obtained in the diphtheria hospital, it was believed, these cases were so little, if at all, contagious, that visiting by the Department Inspectors was unnecessary. Nevertheless, to investigate this question thoroughly, 450 cases of false diphtheria, as nearly consecutive as possible, were investigated, all sources of contagion sought for, and the cases followed up for two weeks after complete convalescence. In none of these was isolation or disinfection enforced by the Health Department. This is such an important question that the results of the investigation of one hundred consecutive cases are given below in tabular form. As a comparison, a similar table is given of 50 consecutive cases of true diphtheria which were taken from the same district and at the same time of the year as the first 50 cases of pseudo-diphtheria.

FALSE DIPHTHERIA.
Table No. 1.

FAMILY No.	CHILDREN IN FAMILY.	CASE No.	AGE.	SEVERITY.	DURATION OF ILLNESS.	MORTALITY.	HISTORY OF CONTAGION, ETC.
			Years.				
1	1	1	4	Mild	7 days..	Recovered.	{ Came from a house where diphtheria was present.
2	2	2	11	"	2 " ..	"	None.
3	3	3	2	Severe ..	30 " ..	"	Complicated by pneumonia.
4	2	4	1½	Mild	5 " ..	"	None.
5	1	5	..	"	....	"	"
6	5	6	8	"	7 days..	"	"
7	3 {	7	6	"	5 " ..	"	} These 2 cases occurred together.
		8	3	"	3 " ..	"	
8	4 {	9	6	"	2 " ..	"	{ These 2 out of 4 children attacked nearly together ; 1 with simple tonsilitis, the other with suppurative tonsilitis.
		10	9	"	5 " ..	"	
9	..	11	..	"	10 " ..	"	Complicated by scarlet fever.
10	2	12	6½	"	....	"	None.
11	3 {	13	3	"	7 days..	"	} The child was first taken sick ; a few days later the servant developed sore throat.
		14	20	"	5 " ..	"	
12	3	15	2	"	8 " ..	"	None.
13	4	16	12	"	4 " ..	"	"
14	1	17	15	"	3 " ..	"	"
15	4	18	2½	"	3 " ..	"	"
16	4	19	9	"	2 " ..	"	"
17	3	20	3	"	3 " ..	"	"
18	4	21	5	"	3 " ..	"	"
19	2	22	10	"	5 " ..	"	"
20	3	23	8	"	30 " ..	"	"
21	2	24	4	"	7 " ..	"	Another mild sore throat in house.
22	2	25	3½	"	2 " ..	"	None.
23	..	26	21	"	12 " ..	"	"
24	5	27	7	"	3 " ..	"	"
25	5 {	28	4	Severe...	14 " ..	"	{ These cases occurred at same time in family. No others developed in house.
		29	9	Mild	2 " ..	"	
26	2	31	1½	Severe...	7 " ..	"	Complicated by pneumonia.
27	..	32	21	Mild	7 " ..	"	None.
28	2	33	25	"	5 " ..	"	Exposed to scarlet fever.
29	3	34	6	"	7 " ..	"	None.
30	..	35	1½	Severe ..	7 " ..	"	"
31	2	36	10	Mild	6 " ..	"	"

Family No.	Children in Family.	Case No.	Age.	Severity.	Duration of Illness.	Mortality.	History of Contagion, etc.
			Years.				
32	1	37	21	Mild	2 days..	Recovered.	Case of true diphtheria in another family in house.
33	3	38	29	"	4 " ..	"	Scarlet fever in family.
34	2	39	7	"	2 " ..	"	None.
35	4	40	2	"	4 " ..	"	Scarlet fever in house one month before.
36	3	41	2	"	9 " ..	"	Scarlet fever in house one month before.
37	3	42	2	"	7 " ..	"	None.
38	3	43	20	"	3 " ..	"	"
39	3	44	30	"	1 " ..	"	The mother, the first case, was never really sick. The child had very slight tonsilitis.
		45	3	"	7 " ..	"	
40	3	46	3	"	4 " ..	"	None.
41	2	47	19	Severe...	10 " ..	"	"
42	2	48	2½	Mild	10 " ..	"	"
43	3	49	6	"	7 " ..	"	"
44	6	50	2	Severe ..	7 " ..	"	"
45	3	51	18	Mild	5 " ..	"	"
46	2	52	2½	Severe...	10 " ..	"	"
47	4	53	3½	Mild	3 " ..	"	Another case in house.
48	..	54	24	"	4 " ..	"	None.
49	3	55	8	"	30 " ..	"	Scarlet fever as complication. Other cases of scarlet fever in house.
50	..	56	2	"	10 " ..	"	None.

Table No. 2.

Family No.	Children in Family.	Case No.	Age.	Severity.	Duration of Illness.	Mortality.	History of Contagion, etc.
			Years.				
1	4	1	8	Mild	2 days..	Recovered.	First case one week previous to second. No others in house.
		2	5	"	5 " ..	"	
2	1	3	30	"	1 " ..	"	None.
3	2	4	32	"	2 " ..	"	"
4	4	5	11	"	6 " ..	"	"
5	..	6	16	"	2 " ..	"	"
6	..	7	19	"	5 " ..	"	Scarlet fever in house.
7	2	8	19	Severe ..	5 " ..	"	Followed surgical operation on throat.
8	..	9	19	Mild	3 " ..	"	Scarlet fever in house.

Family No.	Children in Family.	Case No.	Age.	Severity.	Duration of Illness.	Mortality.	History of Contagion, etc.
			Years.				
9	..	10	2	Severe ..	15 days..	Recovered.	None.
10	7	11	16	Mild	1 " ..	"	"
11	2	12	12	"	3 " ..	"	"
12	1	13	4	"	3 " ..	"	Scarlet fever in house.
13	3	14	2	"	3 " ..	"	" "
14	..	15	3½	"	3 " ..	"	None.
15	5 {	16	4	"	3 " ..	"	{ These 2 children were taken sick together; 1 with mild "croup" and the other with tonsilitis.
		17	2	"	2 " ..	"	
16	1	18	8	"	2 " ..	"	None.
17	..	19	3	"	3 " ..	"	"
18	2	20	12	"	4 " ..	"	Scarlet fever as complication.
19	3	21	6	Severe ..	7 " ..	"	Scarlet fever previously in house.
20	3	22	9	" ..	6 weeks.	"	Scarlet fever as complication.
21	..	23	4	Mild	3 days..	"	None.
22	1	24	2½	"	2 " ..	"	"
23	4	25	5	"	5 " ..	"	"
24	1	26	9	"	3 " ..	"	Measles in house.
25	4	27	20	"	7 " ..	"	{ This and following case occurred in same house one week apart.
26	4	28	22	Severe...	7 " ..	"	
27	4 {	29	6	Mild	12 " ..	"	} These children slept together; 2 had very mild sore throat, while the 3d had a more severe attack, complicated by mumps.
		30	5	Severe...	21 " ..	"	
		31	3	Mild	5 " ..	"	
28	3	32	25	"	10 " ..	"	None.
29	2	33	13	"	6 " ..	"	"
30	1 {	34	4½	"	10 " ..	"	} These 2 cases, mother and child, had sore throats within three days of each other.
		35	26	"	5 " ..	"	
31	4	36	8 mos.	Severe ..	14 " ..	"	{ Complicated by scarlet fever; other cases in family.
32	3	37	5	" ..	30 " ..	"	Scarlet fever as a complication.
33	5	38	9	Mild	1 " ..	"	A sister had scarlet fever.
34	1	39	30	Severe...	5 " ..	"	None.
35	1	40	2	Mild	4 " ..	"	"
36	4	41	37	Severe...	14 " ..	"	None. Suppurative tonsilitis.
37	2	42	4	Mild	4 " ..	"	None.
38	..	43	20	"	4 " ..	"	"
39	1	44	9	"	1 " ..	"	"
40	..	45	21	"	7 " ..	"	"
41	2	46	20	"	5 " ..	"	Complicated by erysipelas.

Family No.	Children in Family.	Case No.	Age.	Severity.	Duration of Illness.	Mortality.	History of Contagion, etc.
			Years.				
42	2	47	1	Fatal....	7 days..	Died	Membranous laryngitis and scarlet fever.
		48	5½	"	7 " ..	"	Scarlet fever from preceding.
43	2	49	2½	Mild	5 " ..	Recovered.	None.
44	3	50	1½	Fatal....	7 " ..	Died	Complicated by scarlet fever contracted from sister.
45	2	51	1⅓	"	7 " ..	"	None.
46	2	52	19	Mild	5 " ..	Recovered.	These 2 cases occurred in same house a few days apart.
		53	30	"	3 " ..	"	
47	5	54	16	"	6 " ..	"	None.
48	2	55	6	"	7 " ..	"	"
49	..	56	15	"	4 " ..	"	"
50	6	57	7	"	3 " ..	"	"

Table of True Diphtheria Cases from the same District as the False Diphtheria of Table "1."

Family No	Children in Family.	Case No.	Age.	Severity.	Isolation.	Mortality.	History of Contagion, etc.
			Years.				
1	5	1	4	Moderate..	Poor	Recovered.	None.
2	4	2	11	" ..	"	"	Previous case four weeks before.
3	1	3	3	Severe.....	Good......	Died	None.
4	4	4	2	Slight	None......	Recovered.	"
5	1	5	10	"	Good......	"	Other cases in school.
6	2	6	3	Moderate..	None......	"	Two days before 2 children in same family died of " diphtheria." At time of culture child was not sick, but developed diphtheria later.
7	1	7	5	" ..	Good......	"	None.
8	4	8	5	" ..	None......	"	"
9	2	9	6	Slight	Poor	"	2 children had just died of diphtheria in family.
10	1	10	2	Severe	Good......	Died	None.
11	4	11	3	Slight......	None......	Recovered.	From case 3, which was in adjacent room.
12	4	12	10	"	Good......	"	None.
13	1	13	8	Severe.....	"	"	"
14	2	14	7	Slight......	"	"	Sent away for safety from family in which there was a case of diphtheria.
15	2	15	4½	Severe.....	"	"	Fatal case previously in family.
16	1	16	1½	" ...	"	"	Servant had just come from case 9, where there had been three cases in family.
17	1	17	2	Moderate..	"	"	None.
18	4	18	5	" ..	Poor	"	Case diphtheria on floor below.

FAMILY No.	CHILDREN IN FAMILY.	CASE No.	AGE.	SEVERITY.	ISOLATION.	MORTALITY.	HISTORY OF CONTAGION, ETC.
			Years.				
19	3	19	9	Moderate..	Good......	Recovered.	{ Two fatal cases just previous to this case.
20	3	20	3	Severe.....	"	"	Other cases in school.
21	1	21	4	"	"	Died	None.
22	5	22	6	Slight	Poor	Recovered.	{ From a candy store. The proprietor's children had diphtheria. This store seemed the cause of several cases in street and a number in a school.
23	3	23	5	Severe	"	"	Previous case in house.
		24	3	"	"	Died	"
		25	8	Mild	"	Recovered.	"
24	6	26	2	Moderate..	None......	"	None.
25	1	27	4	" ..	Good......	"	"
26	1	28	3	Slight	"	"	A case six weeks before in house.
27	1	29	5	Moderate..	"	"	None.
28	4	30	5	" ..	Poor	"	From cases in school.
		31	6	Severe.....	"	Died	From brother.
		32	9	"	"	"	"
29	1	33	1½	"	Good......	"	None.
30	2	34	5	Moderate..	"	Recovered.	From school.
31	2	35	3	Slight	Poor	"	None.
32	2	36	3	Malignant .	"	Died	"
		37	6	"	"	"	From brother.
33	2	38	4	Moderate..	Good......	Recovered.	{ From school, or from a case next door three weeks before.
		39	2	Severe	"	Died	From family.
34	1	40	5	Moderate..	"	Recovered.	From case in school.
35	4	41	7	" ..	Poor......	"	{ This and following case had symptoms of a cold only.
		42	3	No lesions.	"	"	
		43	8	Severe	"	Died	From family.
36	2	44	7	"	Good......	Recovered.	From school.
		45	30	Moderate..	"	"	From family.
37	1	46	2	Malignant .	"	Died	None.
38	2	47	4	Severe	None......	Recovered.	) Had had a previous case one week before in family. Had just moved to new house.
		48	2	Slight	"	"	
39	2	49	3	"	"	"	None.
40	2	50	5	Severe......	Poor	Died	From case 14, originally from school.
41	1	51	2	"	Good......	Died	None.
42	1	52	5	"	"	Recovered.	"
43	1	53	8	Slight	"	"	From case next door or from school.
44	1	54	9	Severe	"	"	From school.

FAMILY No.	CHILDREN IN FAMILY.	CASE No.	AGE.	SEVERITY.	ISOLATION.	MORTALITY.	HISTORY OF CONTAGION, ETC.
			Years.				
45	3	55	7	Severe	Good......	Recovered.	From school.
46	4	56	6	Moderate..	None	"	"
47	2	57	8	Slight	Poor	"	"
48	1	58	4	Severe	Good......	"	None.
49	1	59	:8	Moderate..	"	"	"
50	3	60	5	" ..	"	"	"
	114						

Summary of Tabulated Cases.

	TABLE 1 (50 FAMILIES). PSEUDO-DIPHTHERIA.	TABLE 2 (50 FAMILIES). PSEUDO-DIPHTHERIA.	TABLE 3 (50 FAMILIES). TRUE DIPHTHERIA.
Total number cases.........................	56	57	60
History of contact with other cases..........	7	7	33
No history of contact.......................	49	50	27
Families in which more than one case developed.	5	4*	13
Recovered.................................	56	53	46
Died....................................		4†	17
Cases complicated with scarlet fever..........	4	6‡	..

* Two had scarlet fever.
† Three of which had scarlet fever.
‡ Six others had been in contact with scarlet fever, but never showed any characteristic rash.

We find, therefore, in 113 cases of false or pseudo-diphtheria, occurring in 100 families, that 14 occurred at the same time with or shortly after some other case, and that it is possible to assume the disease had been directly communicated to them. In 9 of the 100 families more than 1 case developed. In these, as in the other 350 cases of pseudo-diphtheria investigated, it did not seem secondary cases were any less liable to occur where the primary case was isolated than when it was not. In this connection, we must remember mild throat inflammations are very frequent, especially in the early spring months, and that it is quite possible where 2 cases occurred in a family together or within a short time of each other, that they may have both been due to exposure to some common conditions rather than to direct transmission. The presence in nearly all healthy throats in New York City of streptococci renders this assumption almost a probability. The presence of the same germs in healthy throats as well as in those of patients suffering from pseudo-diphtheria prevents us from deciding the point by bacteriological examinations.

A good illustration of the difficulty in determining whether these cases are communicable is the following :

In a family of 8 there were a mother, aged forty-five, 6 children, whose ages ranged from twenty-five to ten, and a grandchild, aged two. The family lived on the top floor of a tenement. Two days before being visited by the Inspector of Diphtheria a heavy, wet snow had fallen, which, as the roof leaked, caused the walls to become very damp. The next morning 4 of the children were attacked by more or less severe tonsilitis, which later developed follicular deposits or croupous patches. On the following day the baby had an attack of croup. All recovered, and no further cases developed in the tenement. Here, the exposure to dampness certainly seems to be the explanation of the first 4 cases of tonsilitis, but the occurrence of laryngitis in the baby might with equal justice be considered as due to the dampness, or the result of communication from the others.

Even if further investigation should seem to prove the 14 cases of pseudo-diphtheria out of 113 tabulated, which were found to have had some connection with other mild sore throats, were due to contagion and not to the simultaneous effects of atmospheric or other deleterious conditions, there would still be an important practical objection to sanitary supervision or enforced isolation. All of the 14 cases, except the 3 who had scarlet fever, were mild, and, indeed, leaving out of consideration the cases which occurred as complications of scarlet fever, there was only 1 death in 113 cases of pseudo-diphtheria, and in this case, as has been said, there was no history of infection or contact with other cases.

6. What are the means by which diphtheria is transmitted?

The facts brought out by the investigations of the Department throw important light on the manner in which diphtheria is transmitted.

As related to this question, let us first consider very briefly what is known of the duration of life of the Loeffler bacillus outside of the body.

In actual experiment, the Loeffler bacillus has been found to live for long periods of time, namely: by Hofmann, on blood serum for one hundred and fifty-five days; by Loeffler and by one of us (Park) for seven months, and in gelatine, by Klein, for eighteen months. The bacilli have been found to live in bits of dried membrane by Loeffler for fourteen weeks, by us for seventeen, and by Roux and Yersin for twenty weeks. Dried on silk threads, Abel (26) reports they may sometimes live for one hundred and seventy-two days, and upon a child's plaything, which had been kept in a dark place, they lived for five months.

As examples of the manner in which diphtheria may be contracted, he gives the following from Johannessen:

A teacher developed diphtheria from passing the night in a room in which three weeks before a fatal case had occurred.

A child developed diphtheria after putting on the clothing worn by a child which had died of diphtheria two months before.

In a number of isolated dwellings diphtheria developed nearly a year after previous outbreaks, without there being any apparent possibility of a new infection taking place from the outside.

We ourselves have met with a number of cases where the infected bedding or clothing has undoubtedly been the source of the infection.

4

Sources from which Virulent Bacilli may be Received.

1. From the pseudo-membrane, exudate or discharges from diphtheria patients.

2. From the secretions of the nose and throat of convalescent cases of diphtheria in which the virulent bacilli persist.

3. From the throats of healthy individuals who acquired the bacilli from being in contact with others having virulent germs on their persons or clothing. In such cases, the bacilli may sometimes live and develop for days or weeks in the throat without causing any lesion.

When we consider it is only the severe types of diphtheria that remain isolated during their actual illness, the wonder is, not that so many, but that so few persons contract the disease. This seems to be more remarkable when we observe that in a city like New York the whole tenement-house district, at least, is an infected area. This has become evident from the observations made by the Department.

It has been the practice of the Department during the last year to plat upon a city map the location and date of every case of diphtheria in which the diagnosis had been settled by bacteriological examination. After several months the map presented a very striking appearance. Wherever the densely crowded tenements were located, there the marks were very numerous, while in the districts occupied by private residences very few cases were indicated as having occurred. It was also apparent the cases were far less abundant, as a rule, where the tenements were in small groups than in the regions of the city where they covered large sections. At the end of six months there were square miles in which nearly every block occupied by tenement-houses contained marks indicating the occurrence of 1 or more cases of diphtheria ; and in some blocks many cases (15 to 25) had occurred.

As the platting went on from time to time the map showed the infection of a new area of the city, and often the subsequent appearance of a local epidemic. It was interesting to note two varieties of these local epidemics ; in one, the subsequent cases evidently were from neighborhood infection, while in the second variety the infection was as evidently derived from schools, since a whole school district would suddenly become the seat of scattered cases. At times, in a certain area of the city from which several schools drew their scholars, all the cases of diphtheria would occur (as investigation showed) in families whose children attended one school, the children of the other schools being for the time exempt.

Another fact noted, perhaps as important as the foregoing, was that with the most careful inquiry it was impossible to find any connection with preceding cases of diphtheria in about one-half of the first cases of diphtheria occurring in different houses.

The two following histories are instructive as showing that special conditions, which are largely unknown to us, determine in every individual the occurrence or escape from diphtheria under exposure. Two children in a family were taken sick with diphtheria and removed to the hospital. The servant (who was and remained apparently healthy) went to another family, where the youngest child developed diphtheria a week later. In the meantime, a case developed in the family living in the next apartments. There were in this latter family 3 other children who were not isolated at all from the sick child, yet none of these developed diphtheria.

The child of a man who kept a candy store developed diphtheria ; there were 4 other children in the family, and these were in no way isolated from the sick, yet none of them developed diphtheria ; but children who bought candy at the store and other children coming in contact with these in school developed diphtheria. The secondary cases ceased to develop as soon as the candy store had been closed.

Many similar histories could be given to illustrate the fact that the majority of persons, and even, perhaps, the majority of children, are not ordinarily very susceptible to diphtheria,·and that in addition to receiving the germs of the disease into the respiratory passages they must be in a condition favorable to the development of the disease.

It seems to be generally true that the more malignant a case of diphtheria is the more likely it is to cause diphtheria in others. This may be due to the high grade of virulence possessed by the bacilli, or to the peculiar association of other micro-organisms in the membrane, or to the wider dissemination of the infectious matter through the discharges.

It is also well known young children are much more susceptible to diphtheria than older persons. It is comparatively rare for the parents of children sick with diphtheria to contract the disease, although in nearly every case they must at some time receive the germs into their throats.

CONCLUSIONS.

1. All inflammation of the mucous membrane due to the diphtheria bacillus of Loeffler should be included under the name " diphtheria," and in this report they have been so included. An acute hyperæmia of the mucous membrane caused by the Loeffler bacilli is considered as truly diphtheria as an inflammation with pseudo-membrane or exudate, and a case in which the lesions are confined to the larynx or bronchi as truly diphtheria as one in which the tonsils and pharynx are involved.

2. Under pseudo-diphtheria should be included all inflammations of the mucous membranes, which simulate true diphtheria and which are due to streptococci, or, more rarely, other cocci.

3. The name croup or membranous croup should be regarded as a term merely indicating that the location of the pseudo-membranous or exudative lesion is in the larynx, and not as describing the nature of the disease, whether diphtheritic or pseudo-diphtheritic. In New York City at the present time, 80 per cent. of the cases of " croup " are diphtheria.

4. The examination of cultures made upon solidified blood serum under the conditions insisted on by the Department form a reliable method of determining whether the diphtheria bacillus is present or absent in a throat. For diagnostic purposes, cultures should be made before the pseudo-membrane or exudate begins to disappear.

5. Virulent diphtheria bacilli were apparently in about 1 per cent. of the healthy throats in New York City at the time of these examinations. Diphtheria, however, was rather prevalent in the city at this time. Most of the persons in whose throats they exist have been in direct contact with cases of diphtheria. Very many of those whose throats contain the virulent bacilli never develop diphtheria. We must therefore conclude that the members of a household in which a case of diphtheria exists should be regarded as sources of danger, unless cultures from their throats show the absence of diphtheria bacilli.

6. The bacilli found in the original serum cultures, which in appearance and staining are identical with the typical Loeffler diphtheria bacillus, may be regarded, for diagnostic purposes, as virulent diphtheria bacilli, if the cultures have been made either from throats containing exudate or from those of persons who have been in contact with true diphtheria, for investigation has shown that over 95 per cent. of such bacilli are virulent.

7. All bacilli which are identical with the virulent Loeffler diphtheria bacillus, morphologically, biologically, and in staining by reagents, should be classed with the diphtheria bacilli, whether they have much, little or no virulence when tested in guinea pigs. Bacilli which have entirely lost their virulence rarely, if ever, regain it. They probably are incapable of causing diphtheria, for the 24 cases in which they were found by us never developed any lesions, nor were they the origin of any case of diphtheria, so far as could be ascertained.

8. The name pseudo-diphtheria bacillus should be regarded as applying to those bacilli found in the throat which, though resembling the diphtheria bacilli in many respects, yet differ constantly from them. These bacilli are rather short and are more uniform in size and shape than the Loeffler bacillus. They stain, as a rule, equally throughout with the alkaline methyl blue solution and produce alkali in their growth in bouillon. They are found in about 1 per cent. of the healthy throats in New York City, and seem to have no connection with diphtheria. They are never virulent.

9. One or more varieties, both of streptococci and other forms of cocci, exist in the great majority, and possibly in all, of the healthy throats in New York City. Cultures from the throats in cases of pseudo-diphtheria contain more cocci, especially more streptococci, than those from healthy throats, but otherwise do not seem to differ.

10. The investigations of the Health Department have given striking evidence of the marked difference in mortality between true and pseudo-diphtheria, for while it was 27 per cent. in diphtheria, it was under 2 per cent. in pseudo-diphtheria.

11. The combined clinical and bacteriological investigation of over 5,000 cases has demonstrated clearly the fact that many of the less characteristic cases of diphtheria and pseudo-diphtheria are so similar in appearance, symptoms and duration, that it is impossible to separate them, except by bacteriological examinations. In the more severe cases and after the disease has fully developed, cultures are less necessary, although their systematic use is desirable.

12. Persons who have suffered from diphtheria should be kept isolated until cultures prove the bacilli have disappeared from the throat, for not only are the bacilli which persist in the throat virulent, but they are not infrequently the cause of diphtheria in others. Where cultures cannot be made, isolation should be continued for at least three weeks after the disappearance of the membrane, for our experience has shown that it is not unusual for the bacilli to persist this length of time.

13. In pharyngeal cases in which thorough irrigation of the nostrils and throat with 1-4,000 bi-chloride of mercury solution has been practiced every few hours, the bacilli have not remained in the throat for as long a time after the complete disappearance of the pseudo-membrane as when no antiseptic has been employed. Other cleansing and antiseptic solutions are also useful.

14. Inflammations of the mucous membranes due to streptococci, either alone or associated with other cocci, are usually mild in character. These inflammations may be more serious when the lesions are located in the larynx, or when they are complicated by scarlet fever or measles.

15. While the streptococci and perhaps other forms of cocci may be considered as the primary etiological factor in pseudo-diphtheria, yet, in the majority of cases at least, certain predisposing factors, such as exposure to cold or other deleterious influences or the presence of certain infectious diseases, appear to be of great importance in determining the occurrence of the disease.

The streptococci which under these conditions apparently cause the disease are probably those which had for a long time existed in the throat, and not those freshly derived through communication with other cases of pseudo-diphtheria. In a small number of cases, indeed, the histories suggest a direct communication, but the causation may be equally well explained by the supposition that the second case shared with the original one the same predisposing cause.

16. The slight mortality and the usual mildness of the cases of pseudo-diphtheria do not warrant us in enforcing isolation, even if further investigation produced positive proof that this disease is directly communicable.

With the results of these investigations before us, we can appreciate the difficulty of exterminating diphtheria from a city like New York. On the one hand, we have cases of diphtheria scattered all through the city, many of which are so mild as to be unrecognized, and, on the other hand, we have the crowded tenements with their ignorant and shifting population, where proper isolation of the patient from other members of the family, or of the family from other inmates of the building, is usually impossible unless harsher measures are adopted than are now customary. With stricter isolation of patients and intelligent and systematic supervision of the schools and tenements, we can certainly reduce the number of cases of diphtheria in the city, but the total extermination of the disease under the existing conditions of life here does not seem probable unless we can acquire new means to combat the disease.

REFERENCES.

1. Klebs—Verhandl. des zweiten Congress f. Inn. Medicin, 1883.
2. Loeffler—Mitth. aus d. Kais. Gesundheitsamte, Bd. 2, 1884.
3. Loeffler—Berlin Klin. Wochen, 1890, No. 39.
4. Roux and Yersin—Annales de L'Inst. Pasteur, II, 1888, page 629.
5. Welch and Flexnor—Bulletin of the Johns Hopkins Hospital, October, 1891.
6. Babes—Virch. Archiv. Bd. 119, S. 463.
7. Welch—Medical News, May 16, 1891.
8. Prudden—Medical Record, April 18, 1891.
9. Baginsky—Berlin Klin. Wochen, February 29, 1892.
10. Martin—Annales de L'Inst. Pasteur, May, 1892.
11. Park—Medical Record, July 30 and August 6, 1892 ; February 11, 1893.
12. Janson—Hygiea, April, 1893.
13. Morse—Boston Medical and Surgical Journal, 1894, and Medical and Surgical Reports of the Boston City Hospital, 1894.

14. Prudden—American Journal Medical Sciences, April, 1889.
15. Hofmann—Wiener Medicin. Wochen Schrift, No. 3, 1888.
16. Beck—Zeitschr. of Hygiene, Bd. VIII, 1890.
17. Roux and Yersin—Annales de L'Inst. Pasteur, 1890.
18. Escherich—Berlin Klin. Wochen, 1893, Nos. 21-23.
19. Koplik—New York Medical Journal, August 27, 1892.
20. Welch and Abbott—Bulletin of Johns Hopkins Hospital, February and March, 1892.
21. Abbott—Bulletin of Johns Hopkins Hospital, August, October and November, 1891.
22. Loeffler—Deutsche Med. Woch., 1890, Nos. 5 and 6.
23. Tobiesen—Antralbl. für Bakt., 1892, b'd. XII, No. 17.
24. Fraenkel—Berlin Klin. Wochen, 1893, No. 11.
25. Feer—Mitth. aus Klin. u. Med. Inst. der Schweiz, Heft. 7 (1894).
26. Abel—Berlin Klin. Wochen, 1894.
27. Johannesen—Difterius forekomst i Norge, 1888, page 204.

HEALTH DEPARTMENT, No. 301 MOTT STREET,
NEW YORK, May 4, 1894.

HERMANN M. BIGGS, M. D., *Pathologist and Director of the Bacteriological Laboratory :*

SIR - I have the honor to make the following report on a series of investigations relating to the persistence of Klebs-Loeffler bacilli in the throats of diphtheria patients in whom systematic irrigation with antiseptic or cleansing solutions was employed :

The cases of diphtheria included in this investigation were subjected to three different methods of treatment.

In the first series the nasal and throat cavities were thoroughly irrigated every one to three hours with warm salt solution until the pseudo-membrane had disappeared, then from one to three times daily until the entire disappearance of the bacilli. For irrigation the fountain or Davidson syringe was used.

In the second series, the cases, besides receiving the treatment given in the first series, had their nostrils and throats thoroughly sprayed every three hours (except during the night) with solutions of peroxide of hydrogen, which varied from 25 per cent. to 5 per cent. in strength. The special form of peroxide used was that known under the name of pyrozone.

The third series of cases were subjected to the same treatment as the first, except that solutions of bi-chloride of mercury were substituted for the salt water solution. The nasal cavities were irrigated every eight hours with a warmed 1-4,000 solution, and the throat every three hours with a 1-3,000 solution. Besides this local treatment, nearly all the cases received frequent doses by the mouth of the tincture of the chloride of iron and of alcoholic stimulants.

The following tables show the results obtained by these comparative tests :

Tabulation of all Cases, Showing Day of the Disease on which Pseudo-membrane Disappeared.

	1	2	3	4	5	6	7	8	9	10	11	12	13	14	15	16	17	18	19	20	21	22	23	Total Number of Cases.
Salt water irrigation and Pyrozone spray	..	..	1	2	2	2	2	2	2	1	2	1	2	1	2	1	..	..	..	..	..	..	1	24
Bi-chloride irrigation	..	2	2	1	1	2	2	2	1	3	1	..	1	..	..	..	2	..	..	..	..	..	..	20
Salt water irrigation	1	2	3	4	3	4	5	6	5	4	..	1	1	1	..	..	..	..	..	..	..	..	..	40
Total	1	4	6	7	6	8	9	10	8	8	3	2	4	2	2	1	2	..	..	..	..	..	1	84

Tabulation of all Cases, Showing Number of Days on which the Bacilli Persisted After Disappearance of Pseudo-membrane.

	Before Membrane.	1	2	3	4	5	6	7	8	9	10	11	12	13	14	15	16	17	18	19	20	21	22	Total Number of Cases.
Salt water irrigation and Pyrozone spray	..	..	3	2	1	..	2	..	..	1	2	..	2	1	1	1	1	3	2	..	1	..	1	24
Bi-chloride irrigation	4*	..	3	2	1	..	1	..	1	1	..	..	1	1	..	3	1	..	..	..	..	..	1	20
Salt water irrigation	..	..	1	..	1	..	3	3	5	2	7	4	6	4	1	1	1	..	..	..	..	..	1	40
Total	4	..	7	4	3	..	6	3	6	4	9	4	9	6	2	5	3	3	2	..	1	..	3	84

* In these four cases bacilli disappeared one day before membrane. In those cases treated with bi-chloride irrigation only were cultures taken before disappearance of membrane, while in some cases examination for bacilli were not made for two or three days after membrane had disappeared.

Tabulation of all Cases, Showing the Duration from First Appearance of Pseudo-membrane to Disappearance of Bacilli.

	5	6	7	8	9	10	11	12	13	14	15	16	17	18	19	20	21	22	23	26	29	30	33	Total Number of Cases.
Salt water irrigation and Pyrozone spray	..	..	..	2	..	1	1	..	1	..	1	1	1	1	2	1	1	1	2	1	3	2	2	24
Bi-chloride irrigation	2	..	..	..	1	3	1	..	2	..	1	..	3	..	1	2	2	1	..	..	..	1	..	20
Salt water irrigation	..	..	..	..	1	1	5	..	2	..	2	3	4	9	2	4	4	..	1	1	..	1	..	40
Total	2	..	..	2	2	5	7	..	5	..	4	4	8	10	5	7	7	2	3	2	3	4	2	84

Recapitulation.

	Average Age of Patients.	Average Number of Days of Membrane before Treatment.	Average Days of Membrane in Hospital.	Average Total Days of Membrane.	Average Days of Bacilli after Membrane.	Average from First Appearance of Membrane to Disappearance of Klebs-Loeffler Bacilli.	Number of Mild Cases.	Number of Severe Cases.	Total.
Salt water irrigation and Pyrozone spray.	13 years.	3	6.6	9.6	9.6	19.2	17	7	24
Bi-chloride irrigation	10.5 "	1.6	6.3	7.9	7.4	15.3	15	5	20
Salt water irrigation.....................	7 75 "	2.4	4.5	6.9	10.2	17.1	28	12	40
Total	10.4 years.	2.3	5.8	8.2	9	17.2	60	24	84

In using the pyrozone 3 different strengths were employed, 25 per cent., 12½ per cent. and 5 per cent. solutions.

With the 25 per cent. solution the average time for disappearance of bacilli after disappearance of membrane was 6.8 days, a somewhat better result than with bi-chloride or salt solution ; but it was very noticeable that the pseudo-membrane treated with the stronger solutions of pyrozone lasted much longer than would be expected from the severity of the disease, and certainly much longer than in those cases where the 5 per cent. solution of pyrozone or the salt or bi-chloride solution was employed. Out of 16 cases treated with the 25 per cent. and 12½ per cent. solutions of pyrozone 10 had membrane from ten to sixteen days, while in another quite bad case traces of the pseudo-membrane persisted for twenty-three days.

The average time from first appearance of diphtheritic membrane to the disappearance of bacilli in the 25 per cent. cases was 17.75 days, this not being quite as good a record as that made by the bi-chloride solution, and about the same as that made by the water irrigation. As all the pyrozone cases received, as mentioned before, thorough washing of throat and nose before and after treatment with the spray, the results as shown in the tables would certainly indicate that the addition of spraying strong solutions of peroxide to the treatment with plain water irrigation had no good result. On the contrary, it would seem from the long continuance of the diphtheritic membrane in those cases treated with the 25 per cent. and 12½ per cent. solutions that they acted as an irritant to the already inflamed mucous membrane.

The 5 per cent. solution caused no noticeable irritation. The pseudo membrane disappeared in the usual time, and it would certainly appear to be the best strength (if any) to use for this purpose.

The best results were apparently obtained by the bi-chloride solution in hastening the disappearance of the bacilli and thus shortening the period of necessary insolation ; the duration of membrane being about the same as in those cases where non-antiseptic solutions were used.

Among the 20 cases on this treatment, 1, a boy four years old, developed mercurial stomatitis in quite a severe form, and another showed symptoms of intestinal irritation ; both of them were undoubtedly caused by swallowing the bi-chloride solution during irrigation, as they had not been given internally mercury in any form. Both soon recovered after the cessation of the bi-chloride irrigation.

Laryngeal cases have not been included in this list, as the treatment tried in these cases could have no possible effect upon membrane or bacilli in the larynx. In 6 cases in which these 3 tests were tried, it apparently had no effect whatever, the bacilli being found in the larynx from thirty to forty days after admission to the hospital.

Since the tabulation of the cases in this report was made I have had 2 cases in which the Klebs-Loeffler bacilli persisted for twenty-nine days and forty-eight days, respectively, after disappearance of membrane. These cases received the bi-chloride irrigation treatment as described above until all signs of the bacilli had disappeared. This would make the average number of days for the persistence of the bacilli after disappearance of membrane and the entire duration of the disease about the same in the bi-chloride cases as in those where no antiseptic was used.

The results obtained in the special series of 40 cases treated with plain or salt water irrigation are similar to those obtained in over 600 other cases treated at this hospital in the same manner, and we have found no antiseptic solution which has materially shortened the duration of the diphtheritic membrane or the necessary period of isolation of the patient.

Respectfully submitted,

(Signed)   A. CAMPBELL WHITE, Resident Physician, Willard Parker Hospital.

THE WORK
OF A CHRONIC
TYPHOID GERM DISTRIBUTOR

George A. Soper

THE WORK OF A CHRONIC TYPHOID GERM DISTRIBUTOR.*

GEORGE A SOPER, Ph.D

NEW YORK CITY.

In the winter of 1906 I was called on to investigate a household epidemic of typhoid fever which had broken out in the latter part of August at Oyster Bay, N. Y. The epidemic had been studied carefully immediately after it took place, but its cause had not been ascertained with as much certainty as seemed desirable to the owner of the property.

The essential facts concerning the investigation follow:

THE OYSTER BAY OUTBREAK.

At Oyster Bay in the summer of 1906 six persons in a household of eleven were attacked with typhoid fever. The house was large, surrounded with ample grounds, in a desirable part of the village, and had been rented for the summer by a New York banker.

The first person was taken sick on August 27 and the last on September 3. The diagnosis of typhoid was positive. Two of the patients were sent to the Nassau Hospital at Mineola. The others were attended by capable physicians at Oyster Bay. None of the subsequent cases apparently resulted from the first, although the interval from the first to the last might permit of this assumption. But whether the disease was transmitted from one person to another after the first case occurred was not a matter of great consequence. The most important question was how the first case occurred.

Typhoid fever is an unusual disease in Oyster Bay, according to the three physicians who share the medical practice there. At the time of the outbreak no other case was known. None followed.

The milk supply of this house was the same as used by most of the other persons in the village, all of whom remained well. The cream also was from a source which supplied several other families in the vicinity.

To the first investigators it seemed that the water must have been contaminated. They were unable to ascribe the fever to food, flies or milk, whereas if they could discover that the water had been contaminated they would be able to account for the epidemic.

The water supply for the house was from a driven well said to be 167 feet deep. The well was at a distance of 210 feet from the house, within 60 feet of a

* Read before the Biological Society of Washington, D. C., April 6, 1907.

stable drain, 115 feet from a privy behind the stable, and 224 feet from two cesspools which received the drainage of the house. The cesspools and privy had been cleaned out in April. The house was provided with one water closet, situated on the second floor. This was used by the family. The six servants used the privy. The sewage from the house was carried by a tile pipe to the two cesspools just referred to. The soil is sandy and gravelly throughout this region.

The water was pumped from the well by a gas engine to a covered wooden tank situated 186 feet from the stable and 320 feet from the house. Water ran from this outside tank to an open tank in the attic of the house, removed from the nearest living rooms by a steep and narrow ladder.

Samples of the water were taken and subjected to careful chemical and bacteriologic analysis. They were collected direct from the pump, from the outside tank and from a faucet in the house. There were five samples taken in all. Four were examined by E. E. Smith, M.D., Ph.D., the well-known analytic expert, and the other by D. D. Jackson, Ph.D., director of the laboratories of the New York City Department of Water Supply, Gas and Electricity.

The essential facts concerning these analyses, including condensed statements of the resulting opinions, follow:

ANALYSES OF WATER FROM OYSTER BAY.

1906.	SOURCE OF SAMPLE.	OPINION OF ANALYST.
Sept. 12.	Faucet in house.	"Sanitarily pure."—Dr. Smith.
Sept. 12.	Outside tank.	"Probably safe."—Dr. Smith.
Sept. 13.	Pump over well.	"No evidence of pollution."—Dr. Smith.
Sept. 27.	Outside tank.	"Typhoid from this source impossible.—Dr. Jackson.
Sept. 29.	Outside tank.	"Evidence does not show pollution."—Dr. Smith.

In addition to these examinations, an experimental study was made of the possibility that the typhoid germs might have percolated through the ground to the well from some receptacle of excrement. On September 29 Dr. Smith put fluorescin in the bowl of the water closet in the house, in the cesspools, in the stable manure vault, in the privy vault on this property and in another on adjacent property and in the bowl of the water closet in a neighboring house. He looked for traces of this fluorescin in water from the well, obtained after much pumping, two days and five days later. Six samples of water were collected during this test. They entirely failed to reveal pollution.

Even this thorough work on the water supply did not entirely destroy local confidence in the theory that the water had been the cause of the outbreak. A contamination of the outside covered tank of such nature as to escape detection by analysis was suspected as offering a possible explanation of the trouble. According to this idea the tank, which had been cleaned early in the spring, might have received typhoid bacilli from the cleaners who, perhaps, carried typhoid excreta on their boots. It was supposed that a gradual accumulation of organic matter from the water and dust from the air, aided by the continued warmth of the summer sun, might have led these germs to multiply until at last they escaped to the water and infected the household.

It did not seem to me that the water theory was tenable. The analyses proved that the well was not continuously polluted. The fluorescin tests showed that occasional contamination was not likely. An inspection of the premises and inquiries concerning the way the outside tank was cleaned made it seem unlikely that this tank became infested in the way supposed.

It would have been more probable to suppose that the tank in the house, which was without a cover and accessible to occupants of the house, had become polluted. Such contamination was not without precedent. Had typhoid existed in the house at the time, it was possible that the tank could have become contaminated in this way. But there had been no case. Moreover, inquiry made it seem unlikely that the tank had been visited all summer. It was much more convenient for persons to get water otherwise than by climbing the narrow ladder to the attic. It seemed more probable that the infectious material had been carried to the house by some person or some article of food.

I was led from the proper track for a time by being assured that no person who had had typhoid, at least within many months, had lived in the house or visited it during the whole summer, and by discovering that the family was extremely fond of soft clams. My suspicion for a time attached to clams. It was found that soft clams had frequently been obtained in the summer from an old Indian woman who lived in a tent on the beach not far from the house. It was impossible to find this woman, but I made inspections of the sources of soft clams at Oyster Bay, which showed that they were sometimes taken from places where they were polluted with sewage.

But if clams had been responsible for the outbreak it did not seem clear why the fever should have been confined to this house. Soft clams form a very common article of diet among the native inhabitants of Oyster Bay. On inquiring closely into the question of the food eaten before the outbreak it was eventually found that no clams had been eaten subsequent to July 15. This removed the possibility that the epidemic had been caused by clams. From July 15 to August 27, six weeks, was too long a period for an outbreak of this character to remain undeveloped. The infectious matter which produced the epidemic had been taken with food or drink, in my opinion, on or before August 20.

The supplies of vegetables and fruit were next considered. It was found that the persons attacked had not eaten any raw fruit or vegetables which had not also been eaten by many persons who escaped the fever.

The history of the house with regard to typhoid was inquired into. It was found that but one case of typhoid had occurred on the premises or been nursed there in thirteen years. This case occurred in 1901. Care seemed to have been taken to destroy the infectious nature of the discharges. The case produced no secondary cases at the time. The house had been occupied every summer since without typhoid.

Attention was now concentrated for a time on the first cases to determine whether the infection could have occurred during a temporary absence from Oyster Bay. It was found that those persons who were taken sick at the outset had not been on a visit, or picnic, or, in fact, away from Oyster Bay on any account for several weeks prior to the onset of the illness.

The social position of the persons attacked differed decidedly. Among the first to be taken sick were a daughter of the head of the family and two maid servants, one of which was colored. Following in quick succession were the wife and then another daughter of the tenant and, finally, the gardener who lived permanently at Oyster Bay and had worked on the place for years.

Believing that some peculiar event might have occurred in the family on or shortly before August 20 which, if studied, might give the necessary clue to the cause of the epidemic, careful inquiry was made into the immediate history of the household at this time. The key of the situation was thus discovered.

It was found that the family had changed cooks on August 4. This was about three weeks before the typhoid epidemic broke out. A cook who had been with the family several years had been discharged and a new one employed. Little was known about the new cook's history. She had been engaged at an employment bureau which gave her an excellent recommendation. She remained in the family only a short time, leaving about three weeks after the outbreak of typhoid occurred. Her present whereabouts were unknown. The cook was described as an Irish woman about 40 years of age, tall, heavy, single. She seemed to be in perfect health.

Here was by all means the most important possibility in the way of a clue which had come to my notice. If this woman could be found and questioned, it seemed likely that she could give facts from which the cause of the epidemic could be ascertained.

When, after much difficulty, she was found, this hope was destroyed. No information of value was obtainable from her. She refused to speak to me or any one about herself or her history except on matters which she knew were already well known.

It became necessary to work out the cook's history without her help. This effort has been only partially satisfactory. Her whereabouts for only a part of the time in the last ten years have been ascertained. About two years of time among the last five years remain unaccounted for. In the last ten years she has worked for eight families to my positive knowledge; in seven of these typhoid has followed her. She has always escaped in the epidemics with which she has been connected.

The most interesting features of the other outbreaks of typhoid with which this cook has been connected follow:

EPIDEMIC AT SANDS POINT IN 1904.

In 1904 a well-known New York family on moving to Sands Point, L. I., to spend the summer experienced an epidemic of typhoid which attracted a · considerable amount of attention at the time. The household consisted of eleven persons, seven of whom were servants. The household arrived on June 1. On June 8, or about one week later, typhoid began to appear.

The first person to be taken sick was the laundress. She had entered the employ of this family ten days before for the summer season. Following this case in irregular succession three other persons were taken sick. Within three weeks after arrival, there were four persons, in all, attacked.

None of the family itself was taken sick. No person was attacked who had been long with the family. The new laundress fell ill first, then the gardener who had not come from the city with the family, but worked on the place the year round, then the butler's wife, and finally the butler's wife's sister. The latter was not in the family service, but lived with the other servants in a little house separate from the main dwelling.

The cook had been in the family nine months, seemingly without suffering from typhoid fever or producing typhoid.

The Sands Point epidemic was confined to the house where the servants lived. There were no other cases in the vicinity. None preceded this outbreak and none followed at Sands Point. No doubt could be placed on the diagnosis. One of the cases, that of the laundress, was long and severe. There was no death.

The outbreak was studied by several persons. Finally, Dr. R. L. Wilson of the New York City Department of Health was called as expert to investigate it. Dr. Wilson examined the water supply, drainage and other sanitary conditions. He caused an analysis of the water to be made by Dr. Jeffreys of the New York Polyclinic. It is unnecessary to describe this analysis or the details of Dr. Wilson's careful investigation.

Dr. Wilson's conclusion was that the epidemic must have been caused by the laundress. In his opinion, she had probably been infected before entering this employment. Her case, he thought, gave rise to the others. Dr. Wilson tried to find how the laundress became infected before joining this family, but was unsuccessful.

EPIDEMIC AT DARK HARBOR, MAINE, IN 1902.

In 1902 a severe outbreak of typhoid occurred in the family of a prominent New York lawyer who had just taken his household, consisting of four in family and five servants, to Dark Harbor, Maine, to spend the summer. Seven members of this household of nine were soon ill of typhoid. In addition, a trained nurse was attacked, as it is said, was a woman who was employed to work by the day.

The first case occurred two weeks after the arrival at Dark Harbor, on June 17. The onset of this case was sudden. In just one week another case occurred. Two days later there was a third. The remainder followed rapidly. The only persons who escaped were the cook and the head of the family; he had had an attack of typhoid fever some years before.

All the servants, except the cook, had been employed in this family for one month or more in New York. The cook had been engaged especially for the summer and had joined the family three weeks before it left New York.

The outbreak at Dark Harbor was studied by a number of persons and especially by Dr. E. A. Daniels of Boston and Dr. Louis Starr of Philadelphia. The house was new, never having been occupied before. It has been impossible to rent it since.

Because of its newness, the water supply of the house was not in every way satisfactory. A tank on the top floor of the house had not been cleaned since it was set in place. Until this cleaning was accomplished drinking water was obtained from a spring.

Water was never believed to have been the original cause of the outbreak. Two analyses of the water were made: one at the Massachusetts Institute of Technology in Boston and one in New York. They confirmed the opinion that the water was safe.

It was suspected that the household supply later became contaminated. A pitcher from a room in which the first typhoid case was nursed was supposed to have been filled at an open tank on the same floor, thus infecting the household supply. But the epidemic had already broken out when this event was believed to have occurred. Typhoid fever was scarcely known in Dark Harbor at the time of this outbreak and has been exceedingly rare since. No case immediately preceded or succeeded it.

It was believed by some that the original cause of the epidemic was the sickness of a footman—the first case. The theory was that the footman contracted his illness before going to Dark Harbor, either in New York or on the way. Dr. Daniels was of opinion that the first three cases received their infection in this way at the same time and place.

On making a careful study of the facts, both views seem to me untenable. The period of time which elapsed from the first to the second case was too short to agree with the theory that the first case led to the others. The incubation period required to be covered in the event that the first three cases were infected before reaching Dark Harbor was too long. Beside, for the most part, these three persons had not shared the same food for a long time.

OUTBREAK IN NEW YORK IN 1901.

The history of the cook before going to Dark Harbor is not entirely clear. In 1901-2 she lived about eleven months in one family. Here a laundress was taken ill and removed to Roosevelt Hospital, Dec. 9, 1901, one month after the cook's arrival. This case was seen by Dr. R. J. Carlisle of New York. The diagnosis was positive. The cause of the attack was not, apparently, investigated at the time, and fuller information concerning it has so far been difficult to obtain.

OUTBREAK AT MAMARONECK IN 1900.

My earliest record of the cook's employment is in a New York family which has a summer residence at Mamaroneck, N. Y. In this instance, a young man who made a visit to the family was attacked, his illness dating from Sept. 4, 1900. The circumstances in this case were such as to lead to the impression at the time that the infection occurred on Long Island. He had spent two weeks at East Hampton within a few miles of a fever-ridden camp occupied by U. S. soldiers at Montauk Point. It was thought that he might have been infected from water or by drinking from a cup used by some typhoid patient, or in some other way not known. Inasmuch as the patient lived in the Mamaroneck household for at least ten days before the onset of his illness and, as his supposed exposure to typhoid on Long Island was by no means reasonably clear, it seems to me probable that he was infected by the cook. The cook left within a few days after the onset of this illness. She had been in the family for three years without, apparently, being connected in any way with typhoid.

OUTBREAK IN TUXEDO, N. Y., IN 1906.

Subsequent to her employment at Oyster Bay, the cook went to live in a family at Tuxedo Park, N. Y. She remained there from Sept. 21 to Oct. 27, 1906. On October 5, fourteen days after her arrival, a laundress was taken sick with typhoid fever and removed to St. Joseph's Hospital, Paterson, N. J. According to Dr. E. C. Rushmore, who saw this case, no other case of typhoid had been known in Tuxedo for several years. Excepting the cook, all the servants had been in the family for two months or more. The cause of the laundress' illness was not made clear at the time.

FINAL OUTBREAK IN NEW YORK IN 1907.

When, at last, the cook's final whereabouts were ascertained, it was found that two cases of typhoid fever had broken out in the household where she was employed. These occurred a few weeks after her arrival. One patient, a chambermaid, was taken sick Jan. 23, 1907, and removed on January 29 to the Presbyterian Hospital, New York. The doctor was first called to see the other patient, a daughter of the owner of the house, on February 8. This second case resulted fatally on Feb. 23, 1907, the only fatal case in this whole record.

A period of two months elapsed between the beginning of the employment of the cook and the beginning of the first case of illness in this household. The New York City Department of Health officially investigated the first of these two cases at the time it was reported by the attending physician and, in the absence of evidence to the contrary, ascribed it to the public water supply.

The foregoing records by no means all the cases with which this cook may have been associated. As already mentioned, I have been able to trace but fragments of her history through the last ten years.

There is a remarkable resemblance between these seven fragments. In each instance one or more cases of typhoid have occurred in households from ten days to a few weeks after the cook has arrived or among people who have, within that period, come to live near her and eaten the food which she has prepared.

In every instance the families have been of ample means and accustomed to living well. In each household there have been four or five in the family and from five to seven servants. Four of the persons attacked have been laundresses. Two have been gardeners, permanently attached to the country places where the typhoid has broken out. All but two of the outbreaks have occurred in the country.

The cook has escaped sickness in every instance. In only one instance is it known that she has worked in a family where no typhoid has occurred. This family consisted of two people of advanced age and one old servant.

In all there have been twenty-six cases and one death. Twenty-four of these cases have occurred within the last five years.

ACTION OF NEW YORK CITY DEPARTMENT OF HEALTH.

Believing that sufficient had been learned concerning her history to show that the cook was a competent cause of typhoid and a menace to the public health, I laid the facts concerning the four principal epidemics here described before Dr. Herman M. Biggs, medical officer of health of the New York City Department of Health on March 11, 1907, with the suggestion that the woman be taken into custody by the department and her excretions made the subject of careful bacteriological examination. I had been unable to obtain her consent to any examination.

The department acted favorably on the suggestion and caused the cook to be removed to the Detention Hospital. She reached there March 19, 1907, after a severe struggle in which she showed remarkable bodily strength and agility. At the hospital the cook was placed in charge of Dr. Robert J. Wilson, superintendent of the department of hospitals, and Dr. William H. Park, chief of the bacteriological laboratories of the Department of Health.

Dr. M. Goodwin did the bacteriological work under Dr. Park's direction. It was expected by me that germs might be found in the urine, but more probably in the stools. None was found in the urine. The stools contained the germs in great numbers. Daily examinations made for over two weeks have failed only twice to reveal the presence of the *Bacillus typhosus,* and on these occasions the sample taken was perhaps too small to reveal them. The blood gave a positive Widal reaction. The cook appeared to be in perfect health.

We have here, in my judgment, a case of a chronic typhoid germ distributor, or, as the Germans say, a "typhusbazillenträgerin."

TYPHOID
BACILLI
CARRIERS

William H. Park

TYPHOID BACILLI CARRIERS.*

WILLIAM H. PARK, M.D.
NEW YORK CITY.

The obscurity of the origin of a large percentage of typhoid fever outbreaks led many observers to the supposition that perhaps some saprophytic member of the colon group might change under bad hygienic conditions to the typhoid bacillus.

Further investigation revealed the fact that a small percentage of persons after recovering from typhoid fever pass typhoid bacilli in the urine. The attack of typhoid fever in some of these cases had been a number of years before. Continued examinations showed that these cases were comparatively rare, and it did not seem possible that they could account for all outbreaks of typhoid fever, where one could not trace the infection to those having the disease.

In 1902 von Drigalski and Conradi found typhoid bacilli in stools of four persons who had had no typhoid fever symptoms, but had been in contact with typhoid patients. Soon it was found that a number of typhoid convalescents continued to pass typhoid bacilli for long periods after recovery. Examinations of persons who had had typhoid fever years before revealed the remarkable fact that 1 or 2 per cent. of them were passing typhoid bacilli, sometimes in enormous numbers. The knowledge that the gall bladder had been found infected at operations for calculi suggested this as the source of the bacilli.

A number of autopsies or operations have since been held on these typhoid bacilli carriers and proven this to be the case. Thus, Levi and Kayser reported, in 1906, a case of a woman, 49 years old, who had had typhoid fever in 1903 and made a good recovery. In 1906 the woman died from some other disease; autopsy was held nineteen hours after death. Typhoid bacilli were present in the liver, in the wall of the gall bladder and inside a number of calculi.

Kayser reports that in Strassburg during the year 1904-5 13.5 per cent. of all cases of typhoid were traced to 6 of these typhoid carriers, all of whom were women and gave histories of having had typhoid from one to 27 years before.

A large number of cases of typhoid fever have now been traced to these chronic bacilli carriers. Thus, Lentz states, in 1905, that seven physicians had then reported typhoid cases from bacilli carriers. The first reports the case of a patient who had had typhoid 3 years before, who was known to cause 2 cases of typhoid; the second reports 4 typhoid carriers, who had had typhoid as long ago as 42 years, 15 years, 13 years and 12 years, respectively. To these 4 were traced 12 cases of typhoid. The third reports a typhoid carrier who had typhoid 19 years before, who caused 6 cases of typhoid. The fourth reports a carrier who had had typhoid 1¼ years before, but to whom no cases had been traced; the fifth had a patient who had had ty-

* Read in the Joint Meeting of the Section on Practice of Medicine and the Section on Pathology and Physiology of the American Medical Association, at the Fifty-ninth Annual Session, at Chicago, June, 1908.

phoid 17 years before and had caused 27 cases; the sixth had a patient who had had typhoid 10 years before and had caused one other case, and the seventh reported a bacilli carrier who had had the disease 17 years before. To this last individual 2 cases were due.

Out of 400 recorded typhoid patients Lentz found that 6 retained the bacilli at the end of periods ranging from 3½ to 13 months. Klinger examined the feces of 1,700 healthy persons who had never knowingly had typhoid and found bacilli in 11.

When the bacilli were in the stools of typhoid carriers, Lentz found that he could not get rid of them by any treatment. Their retention is due, he thinks, to faulty metabolism and concomitant chronic disease. Faulty care during convalescence may also be a cause.

He notes the predominance of women who are carriers over men, and especially married women who have borne children.

In most cases, the bacilli are present in great numbers. Lentz suggests that the gall bladder may not be the only source, but that the appendix and the deeper folds of the-intestine may also be involved.

In conclusion, he suggests the following procedures for controlling these carriers. These, as we note later, can hardly be carried out except in special cases.

1. Disinfection of stools.
2. Disinfection of privies.
3. Police notification.
4. Bacteriologic control of stools.
5. Prevention of any occupation in which the carrier is in a position to infect others.

INVESTIGATIONS ON TYPHOID CARRIERS AT THE RESEARCH LABORATORY DEPARTMENT OF HEALTH.

History.—On March 20, 1907, a cook was brought to the laboratory to have the feces and urine examined. The history as developed by Soper revealed the fact that during the past eight years she had been employed in eight families and in seven of these typhoid fever had broken out within a few weeks or months of her arrival. In all twenty-six cases and one death occurred. Just before her removal to the Department of Health two cases had developed in the family where she resided and one patient died. Bacteriologic examination revealed the fact that fully 30 per cent. of all the bacteria voided with the feces were typhoid bacilli. The urine was negative. Careful cultural and agglutination tests showed that they differed in no respect from bacilli obtained from acute cases. The repeated outbreaks occurring after her entrance in families were in themselves proof that the virulence of the bacilli had remained intact. A curious feature of the case is that the woman denies that she ever had typhoid fever.

Treatment.—This woman has now been isolated for sixteen months. Weekly examinations of the stools have usually revealed large numbers of bacilli, but there have been several intervals when for one or two weeks no bacilli could be detected. Treatment by intestinal antiseptics has proved unavailing. Hexamethylenamin in doses gradually increasing from 100 up to 150 grains a day, has been given for a number of weeks with no apparent benefit. Attention to diet and mild laxatives has caused the greatest reduction, but not their disappearance. This suggests that the chief development of the bacilli is in the intestines, although the source of the infection is probably the gall bladder.

The case of this woman brings up many interesting problems. Has the city a right to deprive her of her liberty for perhaps her whole life? The alternative is to turn loose on the public a woman who is known to have infected at least twenty-eight persons.

This case excited so much interest that I decided to

have tested a large number of typhoid convalescents. Eight months ago there was a typhoid epidemic at the Trenton (N. J.) State Insane Asylum. Through the courtesy of those in charge we were able during the past two months to examine the stools from 52 persons who had had typhoid at that time; 2 of these were found to pass numerous typical typhoid bacilli. Their stools were examined four times. One case revealed the bacilli only once, in the other they were present every time.

The stools of 16 persons, who had suffered from typhoid fever in the Long Island State Asylum, were sent us by Dr. Agnew. Two of these persons were found to pass abundant typical typhoid bacilli; they had been well for six months. Repeated examinations have shown the constant presence of bacilli. One of these cases was so mild that the patient was only suspected to have typhoid fever because of the other cases of that disease.

We have, therefore, found typhoid bacilli in the stools of 6 per cent. of the cases examined. During the autumn we examined the feces from a large number of persons convalescent from typhoid fever just as they left the hospital and found bacilli persisted in the feces of about 5 per cent. It was impossible to trace the cases further.

The bacteriologic tests were carried out by Dr. Goodwin and the Misses Noble and Pratt, bacteriologists in the Research Laboratory.

These examinations indicate that the same conditions exist in this country as in Europe, namely, that fully 2 per cent. of persons who have had typhoid fever are typhoid bacilli carriers. A few of these pass infected urine, but most infected feces. Besides these there are numerous typhoid carriers who never had typhoid fever, but through contact with infection became bacilli carriers. Probably at least one in every five hundred adults who have never knowingly had typhoid fever is a typhoid bacilli carrier.

As the majority of typhoid cases occur before the age of 30, the average life of typhoid carriers is fully 25 years, so that we have the somewhat appalling fact that there are at least half as many recovered typhoid cases who are typhoid carriers as there are typhoid cases in any year and that, besides these, there are the typhoid carriers, such as the cook, who have never had typhoid fever.

What can we do under these circumstances? It seems to me that any attempt to isolate and treat on bacteriologic examinations, as Lentz suggests, is impracticable. When we consider that the presence of the bacilli in the feces of these persons is often only occasional, that numerous contact cases having never had typhoid fever would not come under suspicion, and finally, the impracticability of isolating for life so many persons, we are forced to consider isolation utterly impracticable, except as in the case of the cook already described, where conditions increase the danger to such a point that an attempt at some direct prevention becomes an essential.

We must, therefore, as before, turn to the more general methods of preventing infection, such as safeguarding our food and water, not only chiefly when typhoid fever is present, but at all times, for we now know that in every community, whether it be large or small, unsuspected typhoid bacilli carriers may always be present.

DISCUSSION.

DR. HENRY ALBERT, Iowa City, Iowa: A small epidemic of typhoid fever, traceable to a bacillus carrier, occurred in Cedar Falls, Iowa, last fall. It was an epidemic of thirteen cases of typhoid, occurring at about the same time in three families that lived in the same neighborhood. The water supply was first investigated and it was found that these families were using the ordinary supply of the city, the same as that used by a majority of the people. The water supply as the medium of infection having been ruled out, the milk supply was next investigated and it was found that the families in which the cases of typhoid occurred all obtained their milk from one source, and that no other family in the city was supplied from this source. We then investigated more in detail as to the possibility of the contamination of the milk and found that the owner of the cow, who also did the milking, had had typhoid about fifteen months previously, but had not had a sign or symptom of typhoid since, or for more than a year. A bacteriologic examination of the urine and feces of this man was made and typhoid bacilli found in the urine in considerable number. There was no evidence of an inflammatory condition of the kidneys or bladder. We felt reasonably certain that the epidemic was caused by this bacillus carrier. Hexamethylenamin in the form of urotropin was given and in a few weeks the urine was free from the typhoid bacilli. I feel certain that other epidemics I have observed in the past were caused by individuals of this kind.

DR. WILLIAM LITTERER, Nashville, Tenn.: The subject of typhoid carriers is an exceedingly important one. I have in mind a patient who had typhoid fever one year ago. The patient subsequently developed a post-typhoid necrosis of the rib which was operated on by Dr. W. A. Bryan of Nashville. A sinus appeared and a large amount of pus exuded from this wound, something like four or five ounces a day. This condition existed for three months, the patient growing weaker, rapidly losing flesh, and vague pains developed throughout the body. The surgeon requested that I isolate the organisms in said pus and make a vaccine according to the method of Wright. This I did and much to my surprise I found pure culture of the Bacillus typhosus in enormous numbers. I take this to be unique inasmuch as no other organism, such as the pyogenic cocci or other bacteria could be found in this exuding sinus of over three months' standing. I made a comparative estimate of the number of typhoid bacilli in this pus and found that an ordinary platinum loop full contained nearly a half million of bacilli. This case could be rightfully considered as one of a typical typhoid carrier and an especially dangerous one if the discharges from the sinus were not destroyed. Two months' injection with the autogenous typhoid vaccine produced very gratifying results. The patient is much stronger, gaining steadily in weight and there is an absence of the vague pains throughout body. The sinus has almost healed, only about half a dram of pus exuding in the twenty-four hours. Recently I made another bacteriologic examination and found only a few typhoid bacilli and some specimens of Staphylococcus pyogenes aureus. If the patient ceases to improve I intend to make a staphylococcic vaccine and inject this, with the typhoid vaccine. Dr. Park has called attention to the fact that many of these "carriers" have an infected gall bladder, and it has been suggested by some that, in order to cure this condition, a surgical operation would be necessary. It might be possible to try vaccine therapy in curing these conditions.

DR. M. J. ROSENAU, Washington, D. C.: I can not take Dr. Park's place, but feel sure that if he were here he would say that "typhoid Mary" refuses to submit to surgical interference. She is perhaps justified in this conclusion, because the gall bladder is not the only source of the typhoid bacilli that appear in the feces. Surgical interference therefore may not always correct the condition. Sometimes the feces of these carriers contain such large numbers of typhoid bacilli as almost to displace the colon bacillus; it seems that the typhoid bacillus may take up a natural habitat somewhere in the intestinal tract independent of the gall bladder. We have not been able to find a chronic bacillus carrier of this type in Washington.

TYPHOID MARY

Major GEORGE A. SOPER

TYPHOID MARY

By Major GEORGE A. SOPER
Sanitary Corps, United States Army

INTRODUCTORY NOTE BY THE SURGEON GENERAL OF THE ARMY

The appearance of the following article in THE MILITARY SURGEON has a particular appropriateness in spite of the fact that the history of this remarkable woman has been confined, so far as known, to persons in civil life. It is appropriate for a number of reasons.

First, the story, substantially as it appears on these pages, formed an address which Major Soper delivered before the Surgeons of the Sixth Division to which he was attached as epidemiologist in the Army in 1918.

Second, typhoid has been brought under control largely by reason of work done to prevent the very kind of infection which "Typhoid Mary" produced. Investigation showed that a large part of the typhoid in the Spanish American War was due to contact, and the preventive treatment by inoculation which has been compulsory among United States troops since 1911 has been particularly directed against this method of transmission. And in the present war the disease has been combatted not only by attention to sanitation and inoculation, but by examining cooks and other food handlers for the carrier state in order that no person such as "Typhoid Mary" might be allowed to spread infectious material even among those who were immunized against it.

Since "Typhoid Mary" was discovered, the whole problem of carriers in relation to infectious diseases has assumed an immense importance, an importance which is recognized in every country where effective public health work is done and in every army where communicable disease has been brought under control.

The literature of typhoid now contains many examples of the carrier state such as "Typhoid Mary" exhibited; there have been some carriers who have produced more cases, but it is safe to say that it has fallen to the lot of no person to give by example a more striking lesson of the need of personal precautions in the control of disease than has been afforded by this remarkable woman. Her interesting history contains lessons which should be carefully heeded by everybody, whether in the Army or out of it.

M. W. IRELAND,
Surgeon General, U. S. Army.

THIS is the story of the cook who produced a series of epidemics of typhoid fever and was finally discovered and locked up by the New York City Department of Health. Her general history up to that point is widely known, although few details of it can be given by most persons. Her history after her arrest forms a fitting climax to her career.

How she disappeared, produced more typhoid and was caught again, is now set down for the first time.

The great amount of attention which the case has received is due entirely to the natural interest which it possesses. The case has never been exploited for the dramatic elements which it contains, although these fairly crowd one another throughout the narrative. The circumstances of Typhoid Mary's discovery were simply announced before the Biological Society of Washington, D. C., April 6, 1907, in a brief paper. This paper subsequently appeared in a medical journal.[1] Since then no authoritative account of the case has been written. Most of the knowledge which the world possesses of it has been obtained from newspaper accounts of some of Mary's interesting movements since her original arrest.

Many inquiries have been received by me as to the history of Typhoid Mary since her first arrest, and although I have had no official connection with the matter since I brought the details to the attention of the New York City Department of Health on March 11, 1907, I seem to be regarded as the person to whom all such inquiries should be addressed.

It is in view of the scientific and popular interest in the subject which has continued now for more than a dozen years, that the following notes are made, the intention being to review the essential facts and to give notice to Typhoid Mary's movements since she was first taken into custody by the New York City Department of Health.

HER DISCOVERY

In the winter of 1906 I was called upon by Mr. George Thompson, of New York City, to investigate a household epidemic which had broken out in the latter part of the preceding August at the Thompson country place at Oyster Bay. The epidemic had been studied by experts immediately after it took place, and there were a number of typewritten reports upon it, but its cause had not positively been ascertained. It was thought by the owner that, unless the mystery surrounding the outbreak could be satisfactorily cleared up, it would be impossible to find desirable tenants for the property during the coming season.

The essential facts concerning the investigation follow:

Six persons in a household of eleven were attacked with typhoid

---

[1] The Work of a Chronic Typhoid Germ Distributor, George A. Soper, Ph.D. Jour. Am. Med. Assn., June 15, 1907, Vol. xlvii, pp. 2019-2022.

fever. The house was large, surrounded with ample grounds, in a desirable part of the village, among other handsome places, and had been rented for the summer by a New York banker, Mr. Charles Henry Warren.

The first person to be taken sick fell ill on August 27, and the last on September 3. The diagnosis was positive. Two of the patients were sent to the Nassau Hospital at Mineola, and the others were attended by capable physicians at Oyster Bay. None of the subsequent cases apparently resulted from the first. They seemed all to have been original infections. But, whether the disease was transmitted locally or not, the point of interest lay in the origin of the first case.

Typhoid was an unusual disease in Oyster Bay. At the time of the outbreak no other case was known. None followed.

The milk supply, cream, water and other articles of food which might have been implicated were one by one carefully eliminated as possible causes. The drainage was examined and found satisfactory. Extreme care was used in this part of the investigation in view of the fact that there was a firmly settled belief on the part of many persons that the water had become contaminated from cesspools, a privy vault or stable manure pit. Analyses of the water were made independently by two competent chemists and flourescein was used to study the possibilities of underground percolation. As a result of this particular study it did not seem to me that the water theory was tenable.

I was led from the proper track for a time by being informed that the family was extremely fond of soft clams and that supplies of these shell fish had frequently been obtained from an Indian woman who lived in a tent on the beach, not far from the house, and whose supplies of clams were sometimes taken from places that were not improbably polluted with sewage.

But if clams had been responsible for the outbreak, it did not seem clear why the fever should have been confined to this house, because soft clams formed a common article of diet among the native inhabitants of Oyster Bay. On inquiring closely, it was found that no clams had been eaten for six weeks before the outbreak of typhoid, and six weeks was too long a period for an epidemic of this character to remain undeveloped. In my opinion the infectious matter which produced the epidemic had been taken with food or drink on, or before, August 20.

The history of the house with regard to typhoid showed that no case had occurred on the premises or been nursed there, nor was it believed that a convalescent had visited it in thirteen years, and the house had been occupied every summer since then.

Attention was then concentrated on the first case of typhoid to determine whether the infection could have occurred during a temporary absence from Oyster Bay, and it was discovered that no person who was taken sick had been on a visit away from Oyster Bay for several weeks prior to the onset of the disease.

The social positions of the persons attacked differed decidedly. The first was a daughter of the family; the next two were maid-servants. Following this, in quick succession, were the wife, and then another daughter of the tenant, and finally a gardener who resided permanently at Oyster Bay and who had lived on the place for years.

Believing that some event had occurred in the family or in Oyster Bay, which, properly studied, might give the clue to the cause of the epidemic, the immediate history of the household at this time was carefully inquired into. This gave the key to the situation.

It was found that the family had changed cooks on August 4, about three weeks before the epidemic broke out. Little was known about the new cook's history. She had been engaged at an employment bureau which gave her a good recommendation. She remained in the family only a short time, leaving about three weeks after the outbreak of typhoid occurred. Her present whereabouts were unknown.

The cook was described as an Irish woman about forty years of age, intelligent, tall, heavy, single and non-communicative. She seemed to be in perfect health. She was not known ever to have had an attack of typhoid.

Here was by all means the most important clue which had come to my notice. If this woman could be found and questioned, it seemed likely that she could give facts from which the cause of the epidemic could be ascertained. I had seen typhoid spread in large epidemics under circumstances which led me to believe that it should be regarded as a contagious disease, and I had so dealt with it when acting as expert for the State of New York in handling the epidemic of 1,300 cases at Ithaca in 1903,[2] and later as expert of the city of Watertown, N. Y., in fighting an epidemic of 600 cases in 1904.[3]

When, after much difficulty, the cook was found, no information of value was obtainable from her. She refused to speak to me or to anyone about herself or her history, except on matters which she found were already known.

Her former employers gave freely what information they could, but their minds were not wholly free from bias. Nearly all the epidemics which I was inquiring into had been investigated soon after they occurred and had been explained in a different way. The answers to my questions were therefore unconsciously framed so as to convince me that the original explanations were correct.

[2] The Epidemic of Typhoid Fever at Ithaca, N. Y., by George A. Soper. Jour. of the New England Water Works Association, Vol. xviii, pages 431-461, 1904.

[3] The Management of the Typhoid Fever Epidemic at Watertown, New York, in 1904, by George A. Soper. Jour. of the New England Water Works Association, Vol. xxii, No. 2, pages 87-163, 1905.

Curiously enough the greatest help came from a quarter which was least expected. The office through which Mary had secured some of her situations gave me all the assistance which it possessed. This office, conducted in the name of a woman, was really run by a man. For some good reason he did not allow his own name to be known. Whether by aptitude, training, or both, this person possessed many of the attributes of a good investigator. Without his help Typhoid Mary could not have been found.

In passing, it is interesting to observe that nobody who hired Mary seems to have inquired personally into her references. It seems that the names of some of her former employers were available, but it appears not to be the custom of the patrons of fashionable employment bureaus to inquire deeply into the personal history of the servants. Mary always was accepted on the recommendation of the proprietor. He was trusted to run a genuine intelligence bureau and it is but right to say that, on the whole, he discharged his obligations admirably.

The effort to work out Typhoid Mary's history was only partly successful. There were many false clews and puzzling circumstances. The mystery which had at first surrounded her continued and was often completely baffling. Sometimes it was somebody's memory which was at fault—few housekeepers seem to know anything about their cooks, much less recall the food which they have eaten weeks and months ago. Yet this information, in some instances, was indispensable.

Sometimes it appeared that persons were deliberately refusing to tell what they knew. Twice, I think, I talked with members of Mary's family, but I could never be sure of it. Servants who had been associated with her never gave any help.

Try as I would, Typhoid Mary's whereabouts for only parts of the ten years before the Oyster Bay outbreak could be determined with unmistakable certainty. About two years of the preceding five remained unaccounted for. In ten years she is known to have worked for eight families and in seven of these typhoid had occurred. She had always escaped in the epidemics with which she had been connected.

A summary of the principal epidemics follows:

In 1904 there was an outbreak at the summer residence of Henry Gilsey, Esq., at Sands Point, N. Y. The household consisted of eleven persons, seven of whom were servants. The house was rented on June 1. On June 8 typhoid began to appear. The first case was that of a laundress. Following this three other persons were taken sick in succession. None of the family was attacked. The Sands Point epidemic was confined to the house where the servants lived. There were no other cases before or after, either in the household or in the village. The cause of the outbreak was believed to be connected in some way with the servants' quarters.

In 1902 a severe outbreak occurred in the family of a New York lawyer at Dark Harbor, Maine. Mr. Coleman Drayton had rented a cottage for the summer and just before leaving New York to occupy it with his family had engaged Mary Mallon to act as cook. Seven members of this household of nine were presently attacked. In addition, a trained nurse who came in by the day took sick. The first case occurred two weeks after the arrival, on June 17. One week later another case occurred; two days later there was a third; the remainder followed rapidly. The only persons who escaped were the cook and Mr. Drayton himself, and he had had an attack some years before. These two faced together the burden and anxiety as, one by one, every other occupant of the house fell ill. Mr. Drayton felt so grateful to the cook for the help which she gave him during the epidemic that at the end of the epidemic he made her a handsome present of money in addition to her wages, little thinking that the cause of the whole trouble lay at her door.

The Dark Harbor epidemic was investigated at the time and a written report was made upon it. The infection was thought to have been brought to the house by the maid-servant who was the first to be taken ill. It seems that the servants had access to a water tank in the top of the house and it was supposed that this tank became polluted by the first person who was attacked, thus infecting the entire household. How the original case was produced was not explained, but it was assumed with the easy logic which is familiar in many such investigations that it was contracted elsewhere.

Mary Mallon's history before she went to Dark Harbor is not clear. In 1901–02 she lived about eleven months with one family. Here a laundress was taken ill and removed to the Roosevelt Hospital, December 9, 1901. This attack occurred one month after the cook's arrival. Unlike the other outbreaks, the cause of this attack was not investigated at the time, and full information concerning it has not been available.

My earliest record of Mary Mallon's employment is in a New York family which had a summer residence at Mamaroneck, New York. In this instance a young man who made a visit to the family was attacked, his illness dating from September 4, 1904. The cook left a few days after the onset of this illness. It is interesting to observe that she had been in the family for three years without apparently being connected in any way with typhoid before this. It was believed at the time that the young man had contracted his typhoid before he came to visit the family.

Subsequent to her employment at Oyster Bay, Mary Mallon went to live with a family at Tuxedo, New York. She remained about one month—to be exact, from September 21 to October 27, 1906. On October 5, fourteen days after her arrival, a laundress was taken sick with typhoid fever and removed to St. Joseph's Hospital, Patterson. No other case had been known in Tuxedo for several years.

HER ARREST AND EXAMINATION

When at last the cook's final whereabouts were ascertained, it was discovered that two cases of typhoid had recently broken out in the household where she was employed. These occurred a few weeks after her arrival. One patient, a chambermaid, was taken sick January 23, 1907, and removed to the Presbyterian Hospital. The doctor was first called to see the other patient, a daughter of the owner of the house, on February 8. This second case resulted fatally on February 23, 1907, the only fatal case in the record up to this time. A period of two months elapsed between the beginning of the employment of the cook and the first case. There was some doubt about the diagnosis of these cases at the time of my investigation and no opinion had been formed as to their origin. The cook was about to leave the New York house.

It was at this house that I had my first interview with Mary. I expected to find a person who would be as desirous as I was for an explanation of the way in which the typhoid had followed her. Certainly she could not have failed to be impressed by the strange fatality with which the disease had broken out wherever she went. It must have looked as though it was pursuing her. Could she be connected with it in any way? Possibly she had even thought that she had produced the epidemics.

If she were implicated in the outbreaks it was, of course, innocently. I supposed that she would be glad to know the truth and to be shown how to take such precautions as would protect those about her against infection. I thought I could count upon her coöperation in clearing up some of the mystery which surrounded her past. I hoped that we might work out together the complete history of the case and make suitable plans for the protection of her associates in the future. Science and humanitarian considerations made it necessary to clear up the whole matter.

My interview was short. It started in the kitchen and ended almost immediately at the basement door. Reason, at least in the forms in which I was acquainted with it, proved unavailing. My point of view was not acceptable and the claims of science and humanity were unavailing. I never felt more helpless.

The next interview was staged more deliberately. Mary had a friend whom she often visited at night in the top of a Third Avenue tenement. He kindly offered to manage for the meeting and one night, after her work was done, I awaited her with a physician, Dr. Bert Raymond Hoobler, one of my former assistants, whom I had called on to help. We waited at the head of the stairs in the Third Avenue house.

At length Mary Mallon came. Dr. Hoobler and I described the situation with as much tact and judgment as we possessed. We explained our suspicions. We pointed out the need of examinations which might reveal the source of the infectious matter which Mary was, to a practical certainty, producing. We wanted a small sample of urine, one of feces and one of blood. The urine and feces were to be tested for typhoid bacilli and the blood for the Widal reaction. We hoped we could get some information from Mary at the same time.

Indignant and peremptory denials met our appeals. We were unable to make any headway. Mary's position was like that of the lawyer who, on being told by the judge that the facts were all against his client, said that he proposed to deny the facts. Mary denied that she was a carrier. She referred to the Dark Harbor outbreak for proof of her helpfulness and to the gift from her employer there as testimony of the same. Far from causing typhoid, she had helped to cure it. Nothing could alter her position. As Mary's attitude toward us at this point could in no sense be interpreted as cordial, we were glad to close the interview and get down to the street. We concluded that it would be hopeless to try again.

Here my investigation came to an end. It was evident that, although I had succeeded in collecting only fragments of her history, there was a remarkable resemblance between these parts. In each instance one or more cases of typhoid had occurred in households after the cook had arrived, or among people who had come to live near her and eaten of the food which she prepared. In every instance the families had ample means and lived well, as the saying is.

The bearing which wealth may have on the chance of infection may not at once be apparent, but it was taken carefully into account in this investigation. People who live as did the families concerned in these epidemics are almost isolated from infection by their cooks by reason of the fact that nearly everything they eat is subjected to the heat of cooking after it leaves the cook's hands. The heat kills the germs The cook does not cut the bread or arrange the salad or fruit, for example. All such work is done by a butler, footman or waitress, depending upon the manner in which the housework is organized. The cook comes in much more direct contact with the cooked food of the servants; a fact which probably accounts for the relatively larger number of servants attacked in the several epidemics.

Each household had consisted of four or five in the family and from five to seven servants. Four of those attacked had been laundresses, and two gardeners permanently attached to the country places where the epidemics had broken out. All but two of the outbreaks had occurred in the country. The cook had escaped sickness in every instance. In only one case could I find that she had worked in a family where no typhoid occurred, and as this family consisted only of three people of advanced age it is not improbable that they were immune. In all, there were twenty-six cases and one death; twenty-four of these cases had occurred in the preceding five years.

Believing that enough had been learned to show that the cook was a competent cause of typhoid, I laid the facts concerning the four principal epidemics before Dr. Herman M. Briggs, Medical Officer of Health of the New York City Department of Health, with the suggestion that the woman be taken into custody by the department and her excretions made the subject of careful bacteriological examination. I had been unable to obtain her consent to any examination whatever.

The department acted favorably on this suggestion and, after considerable difficulty, during which a number of officers had to be called upon to help, the cook was removed to the Detention Hospital of the Health Department. She reached there on March 19, 1907. She was placed in charge of Dr. Robert J. Wilson, Superintendent of the Department of Hospitals, and Dr. William H. Park, Chief of the Research Laboratories of the Department of Health. Dr. M. Goodwin did the bacteriological work under Dr. Park's direction.

My third and last attempt at an interview was after her arrest. Mary was in a separate room at the Detention Hospital. I explained that I had come to get some information from her. It was desirable to know whether she had ever had an attack of typhoid and, if so, where and when. Would she consent to give a complete history of her experience with typhoid? The information might help many. It could not possibly hurt her. It might prove very helpful in explaining her case. As matters stood, nobody accused her of deliberately intending any harm. If possible, she was to be freed from her disease-producing capacity.

This interview was shorter than the other two. Without uttering a word Mary retreated with dignity to the toilet, leaving me standing alone in the room.

It was expected by me that the germs might be found in the urine, but more probably in the stools. None was found in the urine. The stools contained the germs in great numbers. Daily examinations made for over two weeks failed only twice to reveal the presence of the *Bacillus typhosus*, and on these occasions the sample taken was perhaps too small to reveal them. The blood gave a positive Widal reaction. The cook appeared to be in perfect health.

The feces were examined on an average of three times a week from March 20 to November 16, 1907, and in only a comparatively few instances did the investigators fail to find the bacilli. During the summer months the culture plates contained only a few typhoid-like colonies. In July there were five consecutive negative tests followed by a positive one.

During August the stools showed no typhoid; in September they began to appear again; from September 11 to October 14, 1907, the feces failed to yield typhoid bacilli. During this time the patient's diet was carefully regulated and she was receiving mild laxatives. On October 16, 1907, a very thorough test showed that the germs were again present. From October 16, 1907, to February 5, 1908, weekly examinations of the stools gave, with only two exceptions, from 25 to 50 per cent typhoid-like colonies on the culture plates. These exceptions were on November 13 and December 4, when no typhoid was found.

The implication was plain. The cook was virtually a living culture tube in which the germs of typhoid multiplied and from which they escaped in the movements from her bowels. When at toilet her hands became soiled, perhaps unconsciously and invisibly so. When she prepared a meal, the germs were washed and rubbed from her fingers into the food. No housekeeper ever gave me to understand that Mary was a particularly clean cook.

In the Oyster Bay outbreak, which was studied with more particularity than the others, the infectious matter is believed to have been carried from the cook's hands to the people who were later taken sick by means of ice cream containing cut-up peaches. Mary prepared this herself. In this instance no heat sterilized the washings from her hands.

Mary Mallon was kept virtually a prisoner by the Department of Health for three years. At first she was held at the hospital for contagious diseases at the foot of East 16th Street, Manhattan; later she was removed to Riverside Hospital on North Brother's Island in the East River, between Hell Gate and Long Island Sound. She was employed in various ways, sometimes as laundress. She was allowed to receive friends and enjoyed such privileges as were possible, but she never became reconciled to her detention.

Two legal actions were brought to secure her release. The claims made on her behalf were that she was being deprived of her liberty without ever having committed a crime or knowingly having done injury to any persons or property; she was held without being given a hearing; she was apparently under life sentence; it was contrary to the Constitution of the United States to hold her under the circumstances; such action on the part of the authorities was without precedent. These legal actions were argued with much ability. It was expected that, if she won, she would recover heavy damages.

The case attracted a great deal of public notice, some of the newspapers going to the extent of printing the arguments with illustrations of the unfortunate woman. The courts held that the Department of Health acted within its rights in keeping Mary Mallon in custody and that they were well serving the public interests in refusing to release her.

Public sentiment, to judge by the illustrations, was a trifle mixed. On the one hand Mary was pictured as frying deadly typhoid bacilli the size of sausages in preparation for the family meal, and on the other she was shown sitting lone and dejected on her island with a mongrel dog as her solitary companion. *Punch*, the famous English funny paper, devoted a column of poetry to the case.

HER DISAPPEARANCE AND REDISCOVERY

Although the courts refused to order her release, there was a good deal of sympathy for Typhoid Mary. Whatever could be said of the consequences of her cooking, she had been an innocent offender. She was careless in her personal habits, but so are most cooks. If she was a deadly germ producer, so were thousands of others who were enjoying their liberty. To many persons who did not know Mary it seemed that she ought to be given her liberty.

In the year 1910, soon after a change was made in the administrative head of the Department of Health, Mary Mallon was voluntarily released on her promise not to take employment as a cook nor engage in an occupation which would bring her in contact with food. It was thought that she had learned in three years how dangerous she was and how to avoid infecting people. She was forbidden to cook or otherwise handle the food of others and was required to report periodically to the Department of Health.

For awhile she kept her promise. Then she broke her parole and disappeared. She was lost sight of for nearly five years. I have been unable to learn her complete history during this period, but from the fragments which have been collected, it is apparent that she continued to enact her fateful rôle of typhoid producer. Due to the fact that the woman assumed various names and left little trace behind to indicate her whereabouts, it was not possible to learn all that was desired.

She seems to have produced two cases of typhoid in a sanatorium at New Foundland, N. J., where she was employed in 1914, and another case in New York City in the same year in a small family where she was living under an assumed name with a friend. This, however, is anticipating the end of the story.

Mary Mallon came to light for the second time under circumstances which were the most dramatic of her entire career.

In January and February, 1915, an outbreak of typhoid occurred in the Sloane Hospital for Women on West 59th Street, New York City. In this epidemic there were twenty-five cases; they were mostly among the nurses and other attendants of the institution. The Sloane Hospital is one of the most capably managed institutions of its kind in America, and in its attention to every sanitary requirement is intended to be a model for the teaching of students in the College of Physicians and

Surgeons of which it is practically a part. In his conduct of the hospital and in his lectures to his students, it was the custom of Dr. Edwin B. Cragin, Attending Obstetrician and Gynecologist, to lay his main emphasis upon scrupulous care of the hands. Yet, as Dr. Cragin freely acknowledged, this outbreak was produced by a woman whose hands became soiled with her excrement and who through careless and dirty habits infected the food of the inmates of the institution. Whether she at first used sufficient care and later became indifferent is not known, but it is an interesting fact that Mary worked as cook in the hospital for about three months before the first case occurred.

She knew, of course, the danger and how to avoid it. She knew that she was violating her agreement with the Department of Health in engaging in the occupation of cook. That she took chances both with the lives of other people and with her own prospect for liberty and that she did this deliberately and in a hospital where the risk of detection and severe punishment were particularly great, argues a mental attitude which is difficult to explain. Aside from such behavior as this, Mary Mallon appears to be an unusually intelligent woman. She writes an excellent hand, and the composition of her letters leaves little room for criticism.

She possesses enough skill as a cook to command high wages and has been able to obtain work in the most desirable situations. Surely a mysterious, non-communicative, self-reliant, abundantly courageous person; a character apart, by nature and by circumstance, strangely chosen to bear the burden of a great lesson to the world. If she had learned and been willing to practice what she learned, she would not have had this costly lesson to teach.

Mary Mallon was officially known in the hospital by the name of Mrs. Brown, but she was jokingly nicknamed "Typhoid Mary" by her fellow-servants when the epidemic occurred, for there were some who remembered the published accounts of Mary Mallon's unfortunate experience of years ago. It was this nickname, applied in jest, that led the authorities to find her out.

When genuine suspicion began to focus upon her, Mary cleverly disappeared. Before she could be apprehended, she moved to New Jersey and then to a home in Long Island. She was finally traced to the Long Island house and was forcibly removed to the Riverside Hospital of the New York City Department of Health, refusing to go there without compulsion. She has been held by the Department of Health to June, 1919, without any prospect of again being released.

HER LESSON TO CIVILIZATION

Mary's status after her second arrest has been totally different from that which she possessed after her first. This is true both as to the legal aspects and public sympathy. Whatever rights she once possessed as the innocent victim of an infected condition, precisely like that of hundreds of others who were free, were now lost. She was now a woman who could not claim innocence. She was known wilfully and deliberately to have taken desperate chances with human life, and this against the specific instructions of the Health Department. She had been treated fairly; she had been given her liberty and was out on parole. She had abused her privilege; she had broken her parole. She was a dangerous character and must be treated accordingly.

The total number of outbreaks of which Typhoid Mary is known to be the cause is ten; the total number of cases, fifty-one. Owing to the fact that only parts of her entire history are known, it is probable that the total number of outbreaks for which she is responsible is much larger than this record indicates. It would surprise nobody to learn that she had produced some extensive epidemics.

The case of Mary Mallon is of exceptional interest for a number of reasons. For one thing it illustrates one of the ways in which typhoid and other diseases may be spread without the real cause being suspected. It also shows that we should be slow in arriving at an opinion as to the origin of an outbreak.

It shows how carefully we should select our cooks, and it calls attention in a startling manner to the fact that we ordinarily know very little about them. It confirms the truth of the adage that the more we pay the less we know about our servants.

The Mallon case affords a striking proof of the fact that our food is not infrequently contaminated by excrement. Here lies, perhaps, a common source of infection. Possibly many of the so-called diarrheas and food poisonings which occur may be ascribed to this cause. Some persons and some families seem to be especially prone to these upsets. Is it not possible that what appears to be special susceptibility is really infection from a nearby carrier in many of these instances?

The story of Typhoid Mary indicates how difficult it is to teach infected people to guard against infecting others. Mary had ample opportunity to know the danger which she constituted toward those whose food she prepared. She knew from being told and she knew by experience. She was aware of the penalty which she would suffer if she broke her parole and caused another outbreak. That she could have avoided spreading infection by obeying her instructions admits of no doubt. She knew that when she cooked she killed people, and yet she deliberately sought employment as a cook in a hospital. Why did she do this?

The case is least remarkable for the reason that it was the first of its kind to be worked out in America. It is surprising that nobody had discovered a carrier before. They are now known to be rather common.

Somewhat similar investigations had been made in Germany, and I make no claim of originality or for any other credit in her discovery. My interest and experience in the epidemiology of typhoid had been of long standing. I had read the address which Koch had delivered before the Kaiser Wilhelm's Akademie, November 28, 1902, and his investigation into the prevalence of typhoid at Trier,[3] and thought it was one of the most illuminating of documents. In fact it had been the basis of much of the epidemic work with which I had been connected.

Koch's address was not the only one printed about this time to show that healthy carriers might exist and give rise to typhoid. Conradi and Drigalski[4] had anticipated Koch and it was probably on the suggestion contained in their paper to the effect that with their new culture medium they had found typhoid bacilli in the stools of several well persons that Koch's flying laboratory was sent to Trier and the ground prepared for his Kaiser Wilhelm's Akademic address.

In the Festschrift Zum Sechzigsten Geburstag von Robert Koch, which appeared in 1903, there are several papers on the probable rôle of healthly carriers in producing typhoid. About this time Kayser, Klinger and others were publishing in Arbeiten aus dem Kaiserlichen Gesundheitsmate reports of cases which they found to be due to persons whose condition was much like Typhoid Mary's. Dr. Simon Flexner kindly called my attention to some of these references after I had concluded my work on the Mary Mallon case.

The literature of carriers has enormously increased in all countries since 1906. Instances of carriers causing large and small epidemics have multiplied by the score. The extent of the danger which is to be apprehended from this source and the steps to be taken to meet it have been discussed pro and con until it would seem that the grounds for a common agreement must long since have been reached.

There is agreement as to nearly everything except how to cure the carrier condition. In some cases the germ focus can be reached and removed, in other cases this has so far proved impossible. The trend of thought has entirely changed as to the cause of typhoid fever. Before the rôle of carriers was suspected, water supplies and milk were considered the principal means of transmission. The carrier idea led many to think that here was the principal explanation of the spread of typhoid.

The present thought is that carriers account for a varying proportion of the total typhoid in a region, the exact figure depending largely upon local circumstances. Where water supplies, milk and other common

[3] Die Bekampfung des Typhus—Veroffentlichungen aus dem Gebiete des Militar-Sanitatswessens, 21 Berlin, 1903.
[4] Zeitschr. f. Hyg. und Infect. 39, 1902, pp. 281–300.

vehicles of typhoid can be satisfactorily excluded from the reckoning, carriers probably account for most of the cases.

As a result of research work done in Europe and America, it has been found that from 2 to 3 per cent of all persons who have typhoid fever become chronic germ producers. Carriers have been divided into many classes and groups: some are intermittent, others continuous. A certain proportion permanently free themselves from infection and consequently their power to produce typhoid. Others never become free.

It has thus far been feasible to cure some of the carriers of their unfortunate condition, but there are others who cannot be cured. Experiments at disinfection and even the removal of the gall-bladder, which is generally the focus of the bacteria, have sometimes failed to produce the desired result.

What is to be done in order to protect ourselves from the danger of typhoid carriers? First, it is desirable to discover the carriers. This is not easy. It is most readily done with the help of a good laboratory. The examination of the feces should be made over and over again. Second, carriers must be told of their condition. They must be taught to use precautions against soiling the hands with the excretions. They must be taught to wash their hands frequently: always after leaving the toilet and always before handling food; they must never handle the food of others and they must try to give up the senseless habit of shaking hands.

We should all be careful to avoid eating uncooked food which has come in contact with the hands of persons whose history is not known to us and who may have contaminated the food immediately before our getting it.

Those of us who have had typhoid fever should be examined to determine whether we are carriers. If we are carriers, our families should be inoculated against the particular strain of the typhoid germ which infects us and special precautions should be exercised against the transmission of the bacilli in the household.

PUBLIC HEALTH
IN
AMERICA

An Arno Press Collection

Ackerknecht, Erwin H[einz]. **Malaria In the Upper Mississippi Valley: 1760-1900.** 1945

Bowditch, Henry I[ngersoll]. **Consumption In New England Or, Locality One of Its Chief Causes** and **Is Consumption Contagious, Or Communicated By One Person to Another In Any Manner?** 1862/1864. Two Vols. in One.

Buck, Albert H[enry] (Editor). **A Treatise On Hygiene and Public Health.** 1879. Two Vols.

Boston Medical Commission. **The Sanitary Condition of Boston:** The Report of a Medical Commission. 1875

Budd, William. **Typhoid Fever:** Its Nature, Mode of Spreading, and Prevention. 1931

Chapin, Charles V[alue]. **A Report On State Public Health Work,** Based On a Survey of State Boards of Health: Made Under the Direction of the Council on Health and Public Instruction of the American Medical Association. [1915]

Davis, Michael M[arks], Jr. and Andrew R[obert] Warner. **Dispensaries:** Their Management and Development. 1918

Dublin, Louis I[srael] and Alfred J. Lotka. **The Money Value of a Man.** 1930

Dunglison, Robley. **Human Health.** 1844

Emerson, Haven. **Local Health Units for the Nation.** 1945

Emerson, Haven. **A Monograph On the Epidemic of Poliomyelitis (Infantile Paralysis) In New York City In 1916.** 1917

Fish, Hamilton. **Report of the Select Committee of the Senate of the United States On the Sickness and Mortality On Board Emigrant Ships.** 1854

Frost, Wade Hampton. **The Papers of Wade Hampton Frost, M.D.:** A Contribution to Epidemiological Method. 1941

Gardner, Mary Sewall. **Public Health Nursing.** 1916

Greenwood, Major. **Epidemics and Crowd Diseases:**
An Introduction to the Study of Epidemiology. 1935

Greenwood, Major. **Medical Statistics From Graunt to Farr.**
1948

Hartley, Robert M. **An Historical, Scientific and Practical
Essay On Milk, As an Article of Human Sustenance:**
With a Consideration of the Effects Consequent Upon the
Unnatural Methods of Producing It for the Supply of
Large Cities. 1842

Hill, Hibbert Winslow. **The New Public Health.** 1916

Knopf, S. Adolphus. **Tuberculosis As a Disease of the Masses
& How To Combat It.** 1908

MacNutt, J[oseph] Scott. **A Manual for Health Officers.** 1915

Richards, Ellen H. [Swallow]. **Euthenics:** The Science of
Controllable Environment. 1910

Richardson, Joseph G[ibbons]. **Long Life and How To Reach It.**
1886

Rumsey, Henry Wyldbore. **Essays On State Medicine.** 1856

Shryock, Richard Harrison. **National Tuberculosis Association
1904-1954:** A Study of the Voluntary Health Movement In
the United States. 1957

Simon, John. **Filth-Diseases and Their Prevention.** 1876

Sternberg, George M[iller]. **Sanitary Lessons of the War and
Other Papers.** 1912

Straus, Lina Gutherz. **Disease In Milk:** The Remedy
Pasteurization. The Life Work of Nathan Straus. 1917

Wanklyn, J[ames] Alfred and Ernest Theophron Chapman.
Water Analysis: A Practical Treatise on the Examination
of Potable Water. 1884

Whipple, George C. **State Sanitation:** A Review of the Work of
the Massachusetts State Board of Health. 1917. Two Vols.
in One.

**Selections From Public Health Reports and Papers Presented
at the Meetings of the American Public Health Association
(1873-1883).** 1977

**Selections From Public Health Reports and Papers Presented
at the Meetings of the American Public Health Association
(1884-1907).** 1977